Zero Drop Outs:

The *Qi Masters* Guide to Finding and Keeping Students in Tai Chi and Qigong

Al J. Simon

www.QiMasters.com

Al Simon — Nov 2019

Al J. Simon, Inc., P.O. Box 130, Hillsboro, Oregon 97123, U.S.A.

First Printing, 2019

ISBN: 9781072927099

In This Book

In this book, you'll discover:

- **Why attracting new students and motivating them is so important to Tai Chi and Qigong teachers.**

- The two biggest "student attraction" problems facing Qi teachers today.

- **Your competition used to be other Tai Chi and Qigong teachers. But today, it's Wal-Mart, Netflix, Amazon, and YouTube. How can you compete against these mega-corporations?**

- How conflicting student expectations sabotage your teaching and ruin your retention rate for new students.

- **The three fundamental skills you need to be a successful Qi instructor. (Hint: Most teachers ignore #3, but it is the most important one.)**

- The difference between an "amateur" and a "professional" Qi teacher is not number of students, number of classes, how much they earn, or where they teach - it's this much bigger difference.

- **Three "behavior-set" changes that you need to become successful at attracting new students and keeping them.**

- Why just trying to be a "better" teacher takes you OFF the path to successful teaching.

- **Why you should IGNORE feedback and criticism from other teachers, family, friends, prospective students, and even your current students.**

- A Five-Step Zero Drop Outs Strategy that finds and keeps new motivated students - it all starts BEFORE you ever step foot in the classroom.

- **What brain surgeons, building restoration experts, real estate developers, and wine stewards can teach us about becoming successful Qi instructors.**

- Why it's harder to find students when you try to appeal broadly to anyone interested in Tai Chi or Qigong.

- **The two things all Tai Chi and Qigong students want from their classes, but can't and won't tell you about.**

- The "small puddle" method to finding students and keeping them coming back for more.

- **The "two list" method for finding "pockets" of highly motivated students to attract to your class.**

- The "avatar" method for finding and identifying your ideal students.

- **My single important "planning" step - I don't create a single course, workshop, program, video,** audio, book, newsletter, or even a simple email without doing this step ... and you shouldn't either.

- The biggest change I made that filled my in-person classes - I wound up having to TURN AWAY more students than I could handle.

- **Why calling your class something like "Beginning Tai Chi" or "Beginning Qigong" practically guarantees you will have problems retaining and motivating students.**

- Next steps: The complete "New Course Development Process" that practically guarantees your success with every new course you teach.

- **How to blueprint your course for maximum student attraction.**

- Open-ended vs. close-ended classes - one is better for beginners, the other for advanced students.

- **Should you mix beginners with advanced students in the same class?**

- The importance of matching schedule and facility to the needs of your students.

- **The pre-course step that makes sure your course delivers on its promised benefits.**

- Your course description should NOT be about the course content. It should be about THIS instead.

- How your "pricing strategy" can make it easier to find and keep new students.

- Why charging too little for your courses is just as bad as charging too much.

- A resource you can use to determine the perfect price range for your classes, workshops, and programs.

- List, offer, media, or message - which is the most important part of promoting your teaching?

- The value of students who are "RWA's" when promoting a new course.

- Size doesn't matter - how to build your list of prospective students.

- How to improve the odds of your "broadcast" promotions.

- A resource you can use to develop the "ad copy" for your next class or workshop. You can use it for printed flyers, brochures, or sales letters, or online on your website, in text ads, as a blog post, or as a social media post.

- How to monitor your promotions to improve the attraction potential of your classes.

- What to do when a promotion fails, and the elusive factor of timing your promotions.

Contents

Your Invitation

Want to become a more successful Tai Chi or Qigong instructor, while at the same time learning more advanced material you can teach your students?

We invite you to join us as we explore how to break through to higher levels of health, stress relief, vitality, energy, and power in your Qi teaching and practice.

For support in taking the next steps towards higher levels in your teaching and practice, please visit us online at:

www.QiMasters.com

Al J. Simon

Attracting New Qi Students Like a Magnet

Attention: Tai Chi and Qigong Instructors (and those who want to be instructors) ...

Fill Your Classes, Workshops, and Programs with Dedicated, Enthusiastic Students, **Cut Your Drop-Out Rate** to Zero, and **Attract New Students Like a Magnet** – with this **Five-Step Secret Strategy** from a Hall-of-Fame Master

Dear Qi Instructor –

Most Tai Chi and Qigong classes have high dropout rates for first-time students. Typically, **40% to 80% of beginning qi students <u>quit</u>** during their first three months.

What causes so many students to sign up with enthusiasm, only to quit during the first few weeks or months?

What can we do as teachers to keep new students motivated and engaged right from the start, and to keep them coming back for more, class after class?

As a Three-Time Hall-of-Fame Master, with 35+ years of Qi experience and 20+ years teaching experience, I'd like to reveal to you **a secret five-step strategy** you can use to attract new students to your Tai Chi and Qigong classes, workshops, and programs.

Whether you are a **local teacher** of in-person classes, a **national or international workshop instructor,** or even a **"remote learning" instructor** who teaches by books, videos, and online courses...

... You'll want to arm yourself with this **amazing "Zero Drop Outs" Strategy** to find new students, and keep them coming back for more.

Motivating Students

No matter who, what, where, when, or how you teach, attracting students and motivating is key to your success as an instructor.

It doesn't matter whether you want five students for a local class, five hundred for a workshop series, or five thousand for an online program.

To be a successful Qi instructor, you need to be able to:

- Find new students.

- Motivate them to join your classes, workshops, or programs.

- Keep your current students interested and motivated, and keep them coming back for more.

- Cut down on the number of students who give up and quit.

Being able to attract new students <u>whenever</u> you need them is what distinguishes a highly regarded, successful instructor. It's where many of the more run-of-the-mill teachers struggle. That worry over finding students and keeping them distracts the independent instructor, making her less effective overall as a teacher.

Knowing how to find motivated students – and keep them motivated – is the key to successful teaching in Tai Chi and Qigong.

Motivating Yourself

After all, as instructors, we can't teach effectively if we don't have motivated, dedicated students.

But it's not just students that need to be motivated.

We also need to motivate <u>ourselves</u> as teachers.

Nothing can be more discouraging for us than to start a class with new, enthusiastic students, and then watch them drop out one-by-one. Nothing will demoralize you, sap your self-esteem, and get you to doubt what you are doing more than losing so many promising students in the first few weeks.

Yet, that's exactly what happens far too often in beginning Tai Chi and Qigong classes.

But it doesn't have to be that way.

Imagine starting a new class full of eager, enthusiastic students. Now imagine that class continuing for weeks,

months, even years - with ALL of the original students and without losing a single student.

At the moment, a class with "zero drop outs" might seem like a fantasy. But you can make it a reality, as long as you understand what it takes to find and keep new students.

The Good News is You Can EASILY Learn a "Student Attraction" Strategy That Works Like a Magnet to Pull in New Students!

Hi, I'm Al Simon. I'm a Tai Chi and Qigong master with **thirty-five years of experience,** and a **three-time inductee in the U.S. Martial Arts Hall of Fame.**

I'm also the author of *50 True Chi Stories; To Float Like Clouds, To Flow Like Water; Three Monk Mindfulness; Qigong Self-Massage and Chi Washing;* and *The Four Treasures of Tai Chi and Qigong.*

I've appeared as a guest on both Season 1 and Season 2 of the *Living Energy Secrets* series, as well as BlogTalk Radio's *Secrets of Qigong Masters.* My articles on Tai Chi have appeared in publications such as *Wholistic Alternatives, Natural Health Newsletter, The Empty Vessel,* and *Qi Journal.* And my Qi program was also spotlighted on Shirley MacLaine's *Independent Expression Radio* show.

But most importantly for this book, I began teaching part time in 1994, and full-time in 2001.

I developed what eventually became known as the *ChiFusion™ Tai Chi and Qigong* program between 1996 and

2003, and I became a full time writer and teacher in the early 2000s. It was in these in-person classes where I first discovered these secret strategies for attracting and motivating students.

I'm also known as the "founding father" of online Tai Chi and Qigong instruction. I was the first master to teach online in 2003, and I now have 4,500 online students all over the world. Online sales of my Tai Chi and Qigong programs have topped over $1,000,000.00 (one million dollars).

Today, I run the *Qi Masters* program. In this exclusive program, a number of masters, teachers, and advanced students have come together exploring in-depth what it takes to be a master.

During all of this, mostly through hard work and trial-and-error, I discovered a five step strategy for attracting new students, keeping them motivated, and keeping them coming back for more.

The Power of This Strategy

In my early days of teaching, attracting and keeping students in my class and programs was hit-or-miss.

But this five-step "Zero Drop Outs" Strategy changed all of that. I can say, without a doubt, that this strategy is what has led to all of the honors and recognitions I've received over the last twenty years. That includes my recognition as a master, as well as my U.S. Martial Arts Hall-of-Fame inductions (one of the few Tai Chi teachers to have received that honor).

These days, I don't teach a class, offer a workshop, create an online training course, record a video, write a book, or even send a simple email to my students without using this strategy.

The strategy is that powerful ... and that important.

It was this strategy that allowed me to quit my day job, and become a full-time, professional instructor making my living teaching Tai Chi and Qigong.

Now maybe you <u>don't</u> want to be a full-time instructor.

Maybe you just want to be <u>the best teacher</u> you can be.

This strategy can help you to become that.

It also solves many of the problems you may face in your own teaching. Problems such as:

- Feeling self-confident and ready to teach others, even before you step into the classroom.

- Earning respect and "authority status" with students, if you don't feel like a "master."

- Enhancing your ability to connect with students to make the learning process easier for them.

- Making sure students understand the value of what you teach and how it can help them.

- Learning to be patient with students.

- Addressing special groups of students who might need more attention.

- Creating programs that fit your schedule and lifestyle.

… and much more. All of these teaching skills and abilities are a natural result of the Zero Drop Outs Strategy.

Putting This Strategy to Work for You

This strategy is the EASIEST way I know of to attract the right students to your class, and to keep them coming back for more.

And now you can learn this strategy, put it to work for your own classes and programs, and watch how well it works for you.

Here's the deal:

A while back, I taught the five-step Zero Drop Outs Strategy to my private *Qi Masters* group. For the masters and instructors in the group, I put together a video presentation course that covered the entire strategy.

The feedback on these videos was amazing. I've never had such a response from the teachers and masters in the group.

Well, because the group found these videos so valuable, we've decided to make this strategy publicly available. So we've taken these video presentations and transcribed them into the book you are holding now.

This book will be an invaluable resource to anyone who is a Tai Chi or Qigong instructor, or who is interested in becoming a Qi instructor.

Because of my experience, and the experience of the instructors who've used this approach, I can safely say ...

This book will be the best investment you'll make in your growth and success as a "Qi Instructor" this year.

Look, I know you may have some doubts about all this. I did too, when I first started. But the good news is that you don't have to struggle for a decade - like I did - to figure out how to attract motivated, dedicated students. That's the hard way.

Instead, I'm handing you the keys to become a successful instructor, and it's much easier than you might think.

So if you are a Tai Chi or Qigong instructor ...

... or at least you have plans to become an instructor ...

... and you'd like to make sure your next class, workshop, or program is full of motivated, dedicated students who will keep coming back for more ...

... now's the time to take the first step.

Are you ready? Then let's get started.

Best wishes,
Al Simon
Certified Tai Chi and Qigong Master,
Three-time Inductee into the U.S. Martial Arts
Hall of Fame

The Two Biggest "Student Attraction" Problems Facing Qi Teachers Today

Why is attracting new students and motivating them so important to Tai Chi and Qigong teachers?

Well it may seem obvious, but as teachers, we can't teach unless we have students.

So we need to be able to attract new students to our classes whenever we need them.

That's the first and most important hurdle in being a teacher: developing the skill to create a reliable inflow of students whenever we need them.

But the second hurdle is retention - keeping the new students you attract.

When it comes to retaining students, there are practical considerations here. You don't want to spend a lot of time, energy, and resources to attract new students, just to have them drop out within a few weeks. You want students who keep coming back week after week.

Unfortunately, retention like that is usually not the case with most classes. I'm not certain about your experience as a teacher or as a student, but most of the stats I've seen show a 40 percent to 80 percent dropout rate.

That means within the first weeks or months, usually 40 to 80 percent of your new students will drop out of your class, and maybe out of Tai Chi and Qigong all together.

I remember that very early on in my teaching career, that was my experience. My dropout rate was about 70 percent, and in some classes even worse. I remember one course, back in 1994 when I was new to teaching. I held a 10-week Tai Chi course. The first week, I had 30 students. By the fifth week, the middle of the course, I had 10 students. By the ninth week, the second to last night, I had two students. And by the tenth week, I had an empty room.

That's exactly what happens way too often in beginning Tai Chi and Qigong classes, especially when you are a new teacher.

Student Attraction Problem #1: Competition

Unfortunately, there are two big "student attraction" problems facing Qi teachers today. And the first problem is competition.

Today's prospective students have more options for learning than they've ever had in the history of Tai Chi and Qigong.

We have more teachers of Tai Chi and Qigong now than we've ever had. Prospective students who live in a big city may have a dozen or more places where they can learn in person.

But even if you live in a small town, and you are the only teacher for miles around, you still have lots of competition … from online and from video.

For video, students can run down to the bargain bin at the local big box store and pick up a Tai Chi or Qigong DVD for just pennies these days, or they can order one from Amazon.

Speaking of Amazon, Amazon along with Netflix and Apple TV will be happy to stream them an instructional video for a few bucks, or as part of the fee they already pay every month.

But here's the real kicker.

Students can always pull up YouTube and find Tai Chi and Qigong instructions there free of charge. So with smart phones and tablets, they have a lot of no cost instruction available just a few screen taps away.

As a teacher, how can you compete against all of these options students have for learning, especially the free options?

But it doesn't stop there. It's not just other Tai Chi and Qigong instruction you're competing against.

You're competing against just about every form of exercise they have available to them, both in person and by video.

If they aren't already sold on Tai Chi or Qigong, they may decide to do yoga, or cardio kick, or some other type of exercise. So you're actually competing against every other exercise program out there as well – whether in person, online, or on video.

Beyond this, your final competition is *inertia*. Your prospective students may just decide to do nothing - not join your class, or not take any of their other options, and just stay at home, eat junk food, and binge-watch Netflix.

So with all of that competition, it's actually amazing we ever get <u>any</u> students in our in-person classes.

Student Attraction Problem #2: Expectations

Once we do get a new student, the next hurdle is *retention* - keeping him or her coming back, week after week.

What makes retention so difficult?

Students may have any number of reasons for quitting, but there is one reason that outstrips them all.

And that reason is "student expectations."

Every student walks into your class expecting to get something out of it. Some may be there to improve their health. Some may be there for martial arts, especially if you teach Tai Chi. Some may be there for stress relief, or to develop qi, or for the more meditative aspects.

There may be one of a hundred or a thousand reasons your students are there. But they are <u>all</u> expecting something from attending class.

Interestingly, even students that are there for the so-called "same reason" – such as health, stress relief, or martial arts

– may have wildly different expectations of what's going to happen in the class.

For example, they may have seen another style of Tai Chi or Qigong, and they come into your class expecting your style to be like that. Some may be expecting a few simple exercises, while others may be there to learn more complex forms. Some may expect to practice at home, but others expect only to have to come to class and just do the exercises in class.

But it's not just about what happens in class. Your new students may also have differing expectations of you as a teacher and as a person. They probably have a picture in mind of what a Tai Chi or Qigong teacher is supposed to be like. I guarantee that you won't fit all of the pictures in all the minds of all of your new students.

When students drop out after a few classes, it's almost always because your class, your teaching, or you yourself didn't meet one or more of their expectations.

Now you might lose a few students if they move away, or if their work schedule changes and they can't make your class anymore. But these will be the exceptions.

Most students will quit because of failed expectations.

Of course, it's not possible for one teacher to meet such widely differing expectations. You couldn't even if you wanted to. No teacher can be all things to all students.

Finding the Solutions

So what can we do about the problems caused by competition and conflicting student expectations? Or to phrase our challenge a little more positively ...

How can we attract new students when we need them, and keep our existing students motivated and coming back for more?

This is where the *Zero Drop Outs Strategy* comes in. The five steps of this strategy work together to address the problems of competition and student expectations.

This strategy solved these problems for me, and I know that they will solve them for you. Most teachers can plug these strategies into their existing classes and workshops "as is," without modification. They can start reaping the benefits of having engaged, motivated students right from the start.

As I said earlier, I don't teach a class, offer a workshop, create an online training course, record a video, write a book, or even send a simple email without using this strategy.

But no matter what type of learning opportunity I offer or what media I use to teach, the strategy is <u>identical</u> in all of these cases.

It doesn't matter if I want three students for a new coaching program, fifty students for a workshop, or a hundred students for an online program. It doesn't matter if this is a beginners course in a subject, or an advanced level course for masters and instructors.

No matter what I offer, I use the same five steps, the same way, every time.

I would bet that these strategies will work the same way for you, just as they are.

But of course, you may have certain circumstances that will require you to adapt these strategies to fit. Maybe because of the type of students you're trying to attract, because of the location where you teach, or because of some other factor that I may not even know about, you may need to adapt some of these strategies to fit your circumstances.

But these strategies are "open" enough that if you need to, you can modify them to fit almost any teaching situation you may encounter.

Before we continue here, I should also say that I'm not a lawyer, I'm not an accountant, and I'm not a financial advisor. So you should seek the appropriate legal and financial advice before taking any actions we discuss here. You'll especially want to make sure that these strategies, your attraction steps, and your promotions comply with local laws, which can vary greatly from city to city, state to state, and country to country.

But I should also say nothing here is just theory. All five steps are actions I've actually taken. As a matter of fact, I know some of you reading this book have been my students for years, or even decades. If you've been with me for any length of time, you've actually seen me do all five of these steps in the classes, workshops, and programs you participated in. These five steps may even be why you joined my classes in the first place.

These Steps Give You an Edge

As I said earlier, I learned all of these steps the hard way. It wasn't until much later I learned that these steps are actually commonly known to smart business people. It's just that they are not used by most Qi instructors.

I've taken what I've learned the hard way, and what I subsequently learned from other business and marketing experts, and put it all together in a way that works for Qigong and Tai Chi instructors.

Of course, the fact that these steps aren't popular in Tai Chi and Qigong gives you an edge.

Specifically, it gives you a leg up with some of those competition problems we talked about earlier in this chapter. **You'll be doing something that few other instructors do for their new students.** That will differentiate you from a lot of other teachers, and will make your classes, workshops, and programs stand out.

So if you start doing these five steps, be prepared to become successful. Be prepared to attract the students you want and to have them coming back for class after class with you.

Before we get to this *Zero Drop Outs Strategy* though, we need to talk briefly about "mindset."

Specifically, I have three mindset changes that will help you to put these strategies to work for you. That will be the focus of our next chapter.

Three "Behavior-Set" Changes of Professional Qi Instructors

What makes a "professional" Tai Chi or Qigong instructor?

Is it the fact they make their living from teaching? Is it the number of students they have? The number of courses they offer? Their certifications or credentials? Who they've studied with or what they've studied? How long they've been teaching? Their qi skills? Their teaching skills?

Recently, one of my online students – who is also a Qi instructor herself - asked me why I decided to make teaching Tai Chi and Qigong my profession, and what I have learned as a result of that decision.

Well, it all started when I got laid off from my "day job. "

I had been a software engineer for about fifteen years when the dotcom crash of the early 2000s happened. The company I was working for closed their doors.

Now, I could have gotten another job as a software engineer. But by the time I was laid off, I was burned out. I had grown to hate corporate life. My heart really hadn't been into it for at least a year or two.

So it was time for a change, and being laid off was certainly good motivation to make that change.

At the time I was laid off, I had been practicing Tai Chi and Qigong for nearly twenty years, and I had been teaching the Qi arts part time for about seven years.

At one point during those last few years as a software engineer, I was talking to my boss at my day job. I said to him, "You know, I make six figures as a software engineer and four figures as a teacher. But based on the good I do for people, that really should be reversed."

Well, that stray thought in a random conversation planted the seed in my mind. I began to wonder what it would take to make teaching Tai Chi and Qigong my profession.

What would I need to do in order to earn a six-figure living as a professional Tai Chi and Qigong instructor?

When I got laid off, that stray thought came back to me. I thought, "Well, why shouldn't I do just that? Why shouldn't I just take the plunge, and turn pro?"

Becoming a Professional Teacher

It's been twenty years since I made that decision. In that time, I've learned a lot about what it takes to be a professional teacher.

Being a pro is not about earning a living, number of students, credentials, qi skills, or teaching skills. None of those things distinguish a professional teacher.

Instead, being a professional teacher is more about mindset and approach.

Interestingly, you can be a "professional" teacher and <u>not</u> earn your living this way. You could teach one class of three students each week for free and still be a professional teacher ... if you have the right mindset and approach.

Conversely, someone could teach a dozen classes a week and earn their living from teaching, but <u>still not</u> be a professional teacher - if his approach and mindset aren't right. He could teach international workshops all around the world, or have dozens of courses, books, and videos, and still not be a professional. Because if he isn't interested in developing some of the professional skills we're about to discuss, none of that will make him a professional teacher.

Instead, he's an *amateur* teacher.

The word *amateur* originally meant someone who does something because they love it. If someone teaches <u>primarily</u> because she loves Tai Chi or Qigong, she loves teaching, or she loves both, then she is an amateur teacher.

Now there's nothing wrong with being an amateur instructor. The term is not a put-down. It does <u>not</u> reflect on the quality of her teaching. It merely reflects her **intentions and approach to teaching.**

You see, a professional teacher has a different mindset from an amateur. Think about it this way. An amateur may have excellent Tai Chi and Qigong skills and top-notch teaching skills. But being a professional requires more than qi skills and teaching skills.

Speaking of Mindsets

When we say that there's a mindset that professional teachers have and amateurs don't, we need to make sure we understand what we mean by the term *mindset*.

Too many people think of *mindset* as something they do with their mind. They treat *mindset* as if it were a certain way they should think or feel about something, or their beliefs about it.

That's part of it, of course. But it's more than that. It's also about what you <u>do</u> with that mindset. Having the "right" thoughts, feelings, or beliefs are worthless if you don't <u>do</u> something as a result of the mindset.

Having a professional teacher's mindset is really more about what you <u>do</u>, rather than how you <u>think</u> or <u>feel</u>.

As a matter of fact, trying to change your thoughts, beliefs, or feelings is usually the <u>hard</u> way to go about making changes in your teaching.

It's usually much easier if you change your behavior first, and let your thoughts, feelings, and beliefs follow. So to make the transition to professional teacher, first focus on what changing you <u>do</u>. Change your behavior first, and your mind will follow.

So when we talk about *mindset*, think of it as *motivation to do something different*. To make that point, I sometimes use the term *behavior-set* instead of *mindset* to help us focus on changing what we do.

The Three Skills of Professional Teachers

In a moment, we'll discuss the *behavior-set* changes that Qi teachers need to make in order to become professionals. But first, let's cover three fundamental skills you need as a teacher.

First of all, to be a teacher, no matter what the subject, you need *subject skills*. That is, you need to know your subject.

For Tai Chi and Qigong, that means you have to have the qi skills required in order to teach. You have to know the styles and practices you teach. I think that's an obvious requirement for being a teacher. Now, you don't need to be a master of these skills, but you do have to be able to perform them at a competent level.

Secondly, you need *teaching skills*. You have to know <u>how to teach</u> in a way that <u>your students can use</u> what you teach.

I like to think of teaching skills as having two major parts.

First, you need *an effective teaching model* that you follow in your classes. A teaching model is a particular method you use to present what you teach that produces consistent results for your students.

To support your teaching model, you need the second part of teaching skills, and those are *in-class skills*. These are the skills you use to demonstrate, describe, and explain what you are teaching and get it across to your students in a way that they can learn and practice.

For Tai Chi and Qigong, this means that you need to have an effective model for transferring qi skills to your students, plus the communication skills to facilitate that transference.

So we have *subject skills* and *teaching skills*. But there is a third set of skills you need as a professional teacher.

Those are *client skills*.

These are skills you use in relating to your students - both the students you already have, as well as new or prospective students that you're considering joining your class.

Client skills include being able to:

- Attract new students to your classes.

- Motivate existing students and keep them coming to class.

- Get students to increase their level of dedication and commitment to their practice and to your teaching.

- Communicate in a way that establishes rapport, helps you be persuasive, helps you promote yourself and your program, and helps you attract and reach new and existing students.

So we have *subject skills*, *teaching skills*, and *client skills*.

Let's look at, think about, and get a feel for these three skills as they relate to professional and amateur teachers.

Behavior-Set #1: Put Client Skills First

You might think the difference between a professional teacher and an amateur teacher is about *how proficient* they are at the three skills. You might think a professional would just be *more skilled* at each of these three areas.

While that's often true, that's <u>not</u> the whole picture. It's <u>not</u> just about skill <u>level</u>.

Instead, it's about *priority*.

Amateur teachers generally spend most of their time learning and improving their *qi skills* or their *teaching skills*. They may spend little time, or no time at all, on *client skills*.

You can spot an amateur teacher because he can talk for hours on end about Tai Chi and Qigong in general, or about the specific style he practices. He can also talk on and on about what he teaches or about how he teaches it.

But when a prospective student calls him up to say she's interested in his classes, his lack of client skills betrays him. About the most he can say to the new student is, *"Hey, we meet on Tuesday at 6 p.m. Here are the directions. Now let me tell you about the style we teach…"*

But a professional teacher, one dedicated to client skills, would handle that situation quite differently.

In the end, the professional teacher may wind up having the student come to her class on Tuesday at 6 p.m. She may also give the student directions. But she would get to that point in a conversation a totally different way.

She knows that it's <u>not</u> her qi skills or teaching skills that make her successful. It is her client skills that make the difference in attracting, motivating, and keeping new students.

And those client skills have to be top-notch. All things being equal, that's what distinguishes a professional instructor. It's her priority for developing client skills.

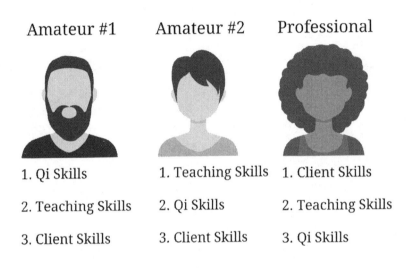

Amateur #1

1. Qi Skills

2. Teaching Skills

3. Client Skills

Amateur #2

1. Teaching Skills

2. Qi Skills

3. Client Skills

Professional

1. Client Skills

2. Teaching Skills

3. Qi Skills

Amateurs put qi skills or teaching skills ahead of client skills. But professionals put client skills first.

So as a result ...

A professional teacher spends most of his or her time as an instructor developing top notch client skills.

Yes, you need qi skills, and yes, you need to know how to teach. But what makes you a professional teacher is knowing how to communicate, how to establish rapport, how to be persuasive, and how to promote yourself and your classes.

What's important is that when it comes to finding, attracting, and keeping new students for your classes and programs ...

Your client skills actually start <u>before</u> a single student signs up for your class.

Since that's so important, let me repeat it again.

In order to attract dedicated, motivated students to your classes, workshops, and programs, you need to put client skills to work for you <u>before</u> a student signs up.

Your client skills start right at the *point of first contact* – that is, when the student first hears about your classes. It happens even before you meet the student and before the student registers. Your client skills go to work when the student first reads about your classes on a flyer, looks at your website, or finds your social media page.

When a student first finds out about you, that's where your client skills need to kick in - and they continue all the way through the registration process.

They also continue <u>after</u> the student joins your program. Those skills are important not just for attracting new students, but for retaining those students and keeping them coming back to your classes.

In addition, client attraction and retention skills aren't just for new students. You need to continue to use them all of the time with <u>all</u> of your students. These skills are just as important with your diehard students who've been with you for twenty years as they are with your brand, new, "first day in class" students.

So that's really the mindset or *behavior-set* that you have to look at first in order to be a professional instructor.

That behavior-set, in just a few words is: **Put client skills first.**

Dedicate yourself to developing client skills as much as you dedicate yourself to developing qi skills or teaching skills.

Actually, dedicate yourself <u>more</u> to developing top-notch client skills, and you'll ensure your success as a professional instructor.

Behavior-Set #2: Be Outstanding by "Standing Out"

Our next behavior-set change is:

Be outstanding by "standing out."

I got this idea from the late Earl Nightingale.

Mr. Nightingale was one of the greatest motivational speakers of the last century. His 1957 recording entitled *The Strangest Secret* was the first motivational, spoken-word recording ever to win a "gold record" for over $1,000,000.00 (one million dollars) in sales.

Mr. Nightingale once said that if you want to be successful, look for role models in your field. Look for those that are having the kind of success you'd like to have, and emulate them.

But if for some reason you <u>can't</u> find a role model like that, then there's another approach.

You simply look at what everyone else in your field is doing ... and do something different. Do what everyone else <u>isn't</u> doing, or what no one else has even <u>tried</u>.

When it comes to Tai Chi and Qigong, you won't find a lot of professional role models. You also won't find many teachers "doing something different" when it comes to teaching.

Too many teachers look, act, and talk all the same. They approach Tai Chi, Qigong, and their classes about the same way as everyone else. They tend <u>not</u> to break out of the mold set by other teachers.

At best, they may look at other teachers and think, "Well, I'll just do what they do, but I'll do it better." That's about the most they'll do. They'll do the same things as everyone else, but just try to be better at those things.

As a result, they become another "me too" in a crowd of "me too" teachers.

Remember what we said earlier about competition? One sure fire way for competition to be an <u>ongoing problem</u> is to make sure you, your classes, and your programs look like every other class or program. When you do that, students will look at you as "interchangeable" with every other teacher.

On the other hand, the easiest and best way to improve your teaching, and especially your student attraction and retention, is to *stand out* from the "me too" crowd.

To be successful, you have to be different. You have to say, think, and especially <u>do</u> things differently from the rank and file of Tai Chi and Qigong teachers.

When you stand out you'll have a much easier time *attracting the right students* to you and *motivating your existing students* to keep coming back to you.

That's the secret right there.

You can become an "outstanding" teacher simply by "standing out" from the crowd.

Here's just one simple example of standing out.

Let's say you're in an area where every Qi teacher posts class flyers on a bulletin board at the local health food store to attract new students.

Well if that's the case, posting a similar flyer on that board is **the last thing <u>you</u> want to do.** Instead, you may want to post your flyer somewhere else – in a place that other teachers haven't thought of.

Or maybe you do use the same bulletin board, but you don't post a flyer. Instead, you put some glossy, professionally printed brochures that your prospective students can remove from the board and take with them.

Or to continue this example, maybe you notice that all the flyers on that board have a class schedule prominently displayed on them. If so, having your schedule on your promotional material is the last thing you want to do. You may want to put on something a little different to attract the right students to you.

You want to do anything you can to make your classes and flyers different from all of the other advertising posted on that board.

You may think that this is a made-up example, but I'm actually speaking from experience here.

In the late 1990's, I was holding a workshop, and I decided to put up flyers in my local health food store to get students for the workshop. Before I made my flyers, I took a look at the other flyers that were posted there. I found flyers for other workshops in Qigong and Tai Chi, as well as yoga and meditation.

But I noticed two things about all the other flyers.

First of all, every single flyer had directions or a map to the workshop location on it. On some of the flyers, a map plus directions took up almost 25% of the page.

Secondly – and remember this was before the internet was popular – none of the other flyers had email addresses on them. They had only phone numbers.

So when I made my flyer, I included an email address along with my phone number.

Now I don't remember if I actually received any email. Email was still new to most people at the time. But here's what's important. Most of the people who <u>called</u> mentioned the fact there was an email address on the flyer. It was one of the items on the flyer that attracted attention. Some asked what email was, since they'd never heard of it before. A few said, "I've never heard of a Tai Chi teacher with an email address."

Because of that, I stood out.

Also, unlike the other teachers on that board, I did <u>not</u> include the map, directions, or even the location of the workshop on the flyer. Every other flyer on that bulletin board did, but mine didn't. Instead, I included one sentence: "Call or email for location and directions."

That "stand out" change had a number of benefits.

First of all, unlike most of the other flyers, I didn't have a map taking up a lot of space. It gave me 25% more room on the flyer to describe the workshop.

I had room to give more details about <u>what</u> was being taught at the workshop – which is much more important than "location" to the dedicated, committed students I was seeking.

That made sure that the people coming to the workshop were <u>interested in the subject</u>. They <u>wanted</u> to be there because of what the workshop was about. And they weren't automatically <u>rejecting</u> the workshop because the flyer said the location wasn't convenient to them.

You can imagine how much better the workshop was when it was full of students who were interested in the subject, and not signing up merely because it was conveniently located to them. To these people, the subject was more important than the location.

It also got people to <u>call</u> me – where I could talk to them and explain about the workshop in more detail than I could do on a simple flyer. That gave me a better chance of engaging my client skills to attract them.

Now that's just one simple example – posting flyers on a community bulletin board.

You may think that's an "old fashioned" example, but the modern equivalent to that is posting class announcements online using social media, classified ad sites, or forums.

But the principle is the same. You need to find ways to <u>stand out</u>, especially when attracting new students. That's even <u>truer</u> today on social media and online classified ads where the competition is more intense.

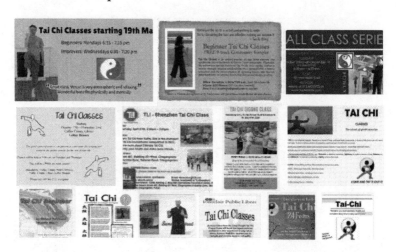

These are some actual ads I found online for Tai Chi classes.

You'll notice that there is a *sameness* to many of these ads. The headlines are similar – usually mentioning "Tai Chi" or "Tai Chi classes." There's often a photo or two. Quite a few use "clip art" drawings. Some even use the exact same clip art figure. And of course, many feature a "yin yang" symbol.

It would be easy to get lost among these ads if you simply post another "Tai Chi classes" ad with photos and yin yang symbols like these.

So here's a simple tip – something you can put into practice right now.

Next time you post an ad anywhere for your classes, <u>don't</u> use "Tai Chi classes" as the headline, <u>don't</u> post photos of Tai Chi, and <u>don't</u> post yin yang symbols.

Post something different.

If you do, you'll have a much easier time attracting and keeping students. They'll see you as different and as someone special - especially when they compare you to the other teachers and programs they have access to.

"What should I post that's different?" you might ask.

That will become clear as we work through the Zero Drop Outs Strategy in the coming chapters. Especially when we get to the fifth step, you'll see one big way you can stand out from all of these "Tai Chi classes" ads.

That's coming up in this book. But before we get to that strategy, we have one more behavior-set change to keep in mind to make sure all of this works.

Behavior-Set #3: Feedback Doesn't Count, Response Does.

Something might happen when you start making some of these behavior-set changes. It will happen when you start putting some of our student attraction strategies in place in your teaching and in your promotions.

You'll find that a number of people <u>won't like</u> what you are doing to promote your courses.

You may get negative feedback from prospective students, other teachers, and maybe even your existing students.

For example, you may hear from prospective students who say, "I would have joined your class, but I didn't like your advertising," or "I don't like what you did in your promotions to try to get me to sign up." They may even complain about how you talk about yourself and your classes, or even the way you talk about Tai Chi and Qigong in general.

You might also get complaints from people other than your prospective students. For example, you might hear complaints from other teachers. They may put you down publicly – especially to their students - for the way you promote your programs and your classes.

You may even hear from some of your existing students about what they <u>don't</u> like about what you're doing to get new students.

But here's an important point:

<u>None</u> of this feedback counts.

When you are a teacher, feedback about your promotional strategies has almost <u>no</u> value. By feedback I mean what people <u>say</u> or <u>think</u> about you, your teaching, or your promotional activities.

Instead ...

What counts is <u>not</u> feedback, but <u>response</u>.

By *response,* I mean what others <u>do</u> as a result of your promotional activities. That's what you're looking for.

As a simple example, let's say you wanted ten new students for a class you were starting. You ran a promotion, and from that promotion, you got the ten new students you wanted. That is a successful promotion.

It doesn't matter if in the process of getting those ten new students, you got complaints from one hundred other prospective students about your new course. It doesn't matter if all one hundred called, emailed, or messaged you, specifically to tell you how much they hated what you said in your promotion.

Those one hundred people who didn't register don't matter. What matters is that you wanted ten new students, and you <u>got</u> ten new students. That makes your promotion successful. And if most or all of those ten stay around and keep coming back month after month to your classes, you can consider your promotion an even bigger success.

So when you promote your courses and programs, pay attention to actual responses and to getting the results you want. That's all that matters.

Ignore any feedback (what people say, think, or feel) and pay attention to what they do.

Let me point out some especially toxic sources of feedback you need to ignore.

Feedback from Non-Students

One source of toxic feedback is "non-students" - the prospective students that saw your promotion and then didn't register for your offering.

Listening to their feedback will mess you up more than anything else.

If you had a successful promotion, if it reached its goals, if you got the students you wanted, then you really need to ignore the feedback you got from non-students.

You'll often find that non-students - the ones that didn't register – are more often than not merely trying to justify their decision not to register. Their criticism isn't serious. It's just their way of rationalizing their decision not to join.

Actually, negative feedback from non-students is often a sign that your promotion was especially "attractive." You were so persuasive that they had to come up with a justification for <u>not</u> registering. Criticism is often a "go-to" method of justification in the face of persuasion.

So more often than not, you won't be able to satisfy these complainers. You'll often find that if you actually try to do something to satisfy their complaints, they <u>still</u> won't sign up. Or they'll sign up, but they become retention problems. They find more things to complain about once they are in the class in order to justify dropping out at a later date.

I'm speaking from experience here. I made this mistake of trying to satisfy complaining non-students more times than I care to admit to. I can't say it never works – occasionally a complainer becomes a good student – but it's rarely worth the time and energy it takes.

And, of course, not every non-student is this way. But it happens often enough that you'll make your "student attraction" a lot more efficient and effective if you ignore feedback you get from non-students.

Feedback from Other Teachers

Another source of toxic feedback is other teachers. They can be an especially toxic source. They may put you down, even publicly ridicule you, when you start *standing out* from the crowd of teachers that <u>they</u> belong to.

Have you heard the phrase "crab mentality"?

It refers to a type of behavior that's been observed when a bunch of crabs are put into a small pot. Certainly, any of the crabs could climb up to escape from the small pot. But often when one crab tries to escape, the other crabs pull him back down into the pot with them.

Unfortunately, a lot of teachers have that crab mentality.

So you need to keep one thing in mind. These teachers are <u>not</u> your prospective students. Your teaching and promotions were not intended for them. So their feedback has no value, since they were not the intended audience.

If you actually try to do something about their feedback, you'll find yourself dragged right back down into their *pot of sameness.*

Remember: it's only the response from those who are <u>right</u> for your teaching and who <u>take action</u> that counts.

Feedback from Friends and Family

There's a third group whose feedback is toxic, and I'm sorry to have to include this group. But often you'll get negative feedback from well-meaning, but misguided "others" in your life – such as family and friends.

They often judge you, your teaching, and especially your promotions from their own perspective. They'll judge them from how <u>they</u> would respond (or not respond) to your promotions. Or they'll respond based on how they think your promotion makes <u>them</u> look because of their association with you.

The truth is though that <u>few</u> of your family and friends are your prospective students.

They are not the people who you are trying to get into your classes. In other words, they are also non-students. So, of course, they may respond negatively, since your teaching and promotion isn't aimed at them.

So don't let their feedback derail you either. Keep focused on the response you are getting from those students you <u>are</u> trying to attract.

Are you seeing a pattern here? Complaining prospects, other teachers, family, friends – they are the people who may respond negatively to your student attraction attempts.

That's because these are the people you are <u>not</u> trying to attract. Your promotions aren't for them. They are all "non-students."

You Are A Non-Student Too

But there's one final "non-student" source of feedback you'll need to be aware of.

And it's a particularly toxic source.

That toxic "non-student" source is <u>your own</u> thoughts, feelings, and beliefs.

As you begin putting client skills first, and as you work on being outstanding by standing out, you may do some things that will make you feel uncomfortable. Especially as we work our way through the five step strategy covered in this book, you may find that some of the strategies are out of your comfort zone.

Just remember: you are <u>not</u> your student. When it comes to attracting students, you yourself are a *non-student*. You are <u>not</u> trying to promote your courses in a way that would attract you. You are trying to promote your courses in a way that attracts <u>your ideal students</u>.

So be prepared for your doing promotions that will make you feel a bit uncomfortable.

As you explore this more deeply, you'll find that feeling <u>uncomfortable</u> about your promotions is a <u>positive</u> sign.

It means you're breaking through the thoughts, beliefs, and emotional reactions that are holding you back from being an outstanding ("standing-out") instructor.

Just remember the advice I gave earlier. Don't focus on changing any thoughts, beliefs, or feelings that are in the way. Acknowledge them, but focus more on what you <u>do</u> than on how you feel about what you do.

Do these five steps, and as you see the results they bring, your thoughts and emotions will catch up to your actions.

Action Items

Note: At the end of most chapters, you'll find one or more *action items*. To get the most out of your new "student attraction" approach to teaching, **make sure you complete these action items before moving on to the next chapter.**

Action Items for "Behavior Sets"

- Memorize the three behavior-sets described in this chapter. They are:

  1. Put client skills first.

  2. Be outstanding by "standing out".

  3. Feedback doesn't count, response does.

- Explain each of the three "behavior-sets" in your own words.

The Zero Drop Outs Strategy

In this chapter, we'll briefly go over the *Zero Drop Outs Strategy* you can use to find and keep new students in Tai Chi and Qigong. The five steps of this strategy encompass the primary client skills you'll need to attract and retain motivated, dedicated students.

Of course, these aren't the only client skills you'll need to be a successful Qi instructor. You'll also need skills in communication, in building rapport, and in other areas of teaching.

Most of those skills, however, don't "kick in" until <u>after</u> you've attracted new students.

So the five skills that we'll be focusing on in this book happen <u>before</u> you start teaching. Actually, they happen before you even offer a new class, or try to reach out to new students.

These five skills - done long before you start a new class - will give you a huge advantage in dealing with the two big "student attraction" problems we mentioned earlier, competition and conflicting student expectations.

Avoiding the Struggle

I mentioned earlier that I learned this strategy the hard way. When I began as a teacher in 1994, I didn't have a business or marketing background.

43

Yes, I had worked _for_ businesses. But I had been a software engineer, and I didn't know anything about the promotional aspects of business.

I also didn't know how to promote Tai Chi, Qigong, myself or my teaching. As a result, I learned these steps by trial and error. It took me a while to figure this all out.

I started teaching in 1994, but I really didn't start figuring this out until about 2003 or 2004. So I spent a decade struggling to find the right way to attract students. Eventually though, I came up with a good chunk of these five steps on my own through trial and error.

Around 2007 or so, I learned that the steps I came up with are actually common steps used by smart business people in an area called _niche marketing_. The five steps I came up with are common among niche marketers.

Since I had figured these steps out on my own, I hadn't learned them in the right order. Also, my original versions of each of the steps weren't as refined as they are now.

Once I started learning about niche marketing, and combined it with what I'd learned the hard way, the whole picture of promoting my teaching fit together. It made all of these steps much easier to do.

Order and Timing

By the way, the order is actually important in performing these five steps. So is timing. As I said earlier, ideally you would use this Zero Drop Outs Strategy before you ever set foot in a classroom. If you have this strategy in place from the start, you'll be successful right from the start. You won't have to struggle for a decade like I did.

But it's never too late to put this strategy to work for you.

You can have it in place before you start your next new workshop, class, or session. If you create books, videos, or online courses, you could put the strategy in place for your next release. It will make it much easier to attract students to whatever programs you have coming up.

You can do these five steps to attract <u>new</u> students, but this strategy also helps you with <u>existing</u> courses and with your current students as well.

So without further ado, let me give you the five steps. I'm just going to list them here. Then, throughout the rest of the book, we'll go into the details and subtleties of each one.

Here is our five-step, Zero Drop Outs Strategy:

1. Find your teaching niches.

2. Identify your ideal students.

3. Find out where those students are.

4. Find out what those students want.

5. Make sure those students know why they should be your students.

Finding Your Teaching Niches

Let's try a little "thought experiment."

I'm going to name several pairs of people with various professions. For each pair, I'd like you to think about and answer this question:

Which one of the two people is often thought of as more skilled, held in higher regard, and felt to be more successful?

That's it. Just that one question.

Ready?

Here's our first pair:

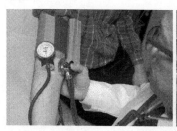 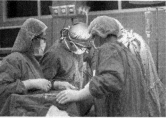

1. A family doctor in general practice.

2. The brain surgeon specializing in seizure disorders.

Which of these two is thought of as more skilled, held in higher regard, and felt to be more successful?

Or how about this pair:

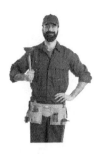 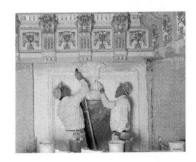

1. A handyman who works around your house for a few bucks an hour.

2. The restoration expert who specializes in restoring damaged historic buildings to their former glory.

Again, which of these two is more successful? Which is held in higher regard? Which is more skilled?

Here's our third pair:

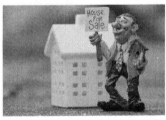 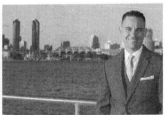

1. A real estate agent for family homes in the suburbs

2. The developer and designer of skyscrapers and large commercial buildings in a major city

Who is more skilled, held in higher esteem, or thought to be more successful?

Here's one final pair for our thought experiment:

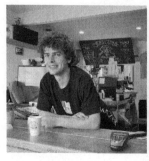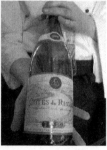

1. An order taker at your local coffee shop.

2. The sommelier (wine steward) at a five-star restaurant who has a detailed knowledge of vintages and of pairings of wine with food.

Which one of our final pair is thought of as more skilled, held in higher regard, and felt to be more successful?

Specialists vs. Generalists

If you are like most people that complete this thought experiment, you picked the second person in each of these pairs. The second person is often seen as more skilled, thought of as more successful, and held in higher regard.

This is not to put down family doctors, handymen, real estate agents, or coffee shop workers.

It's just that those who specialize in a more narrow field of study – like a brain surgeon or a wine sommelier - are often perceived as more skilled, held in higher regard, and more successful.

This is true in every field. The specialist is often held in higher regard.

But what makes someone a specialist? Is it education? Experience? Skill level? Responsibility level? Amount of success? Income? Fame?

A specialist might have some or all of those qualities, but what makes them a specialist is more basic.

It's the types of problems they solve for others or the curiosities they can help others explore.

Someone who solves more specific or more difficult problems, or who has specialized knowledge in an area of curiosity, is often more highly regarded – especially by people who <u>have</u> that problem or curiosity.

As a result, this "high regard" generates a lot of "authority" and "expert status" when it comes to interacting with new clients.

For example, if you are a family doctor, and you say to a new patient, "Hey, you should lose some weight," – well, that patient may or may not lose weight. In some cases, even bringing the topic up will cause the patient to be dissatisfied with you. The patient may even decide to look for another doctor.

But if you are a brain surgeon, and you say to a patient, "We really need to operate this afternoon to save your life," most patients won't leave the hospital to go find another surgeon to tell them what they want to hear. They'll accept your diagnosis because of your expertise.

As a Tai Chi or Qigong teacher, you want to develop the same level of "authority" and "expert status" that brain surgeons have.

Doing so makes it much easier to attract new students and keep them coming back to your programs if they see you as an expert. You'll have a much easier time at getting students than more "generalist" Qi teachers.

So how do we acquire this authority? We do it the same way that brain surgeons, wine sommeliers, commercial real estate developers, and restoration experts do.

The _easiest way_ to acquire this expert status is to _specialize_ in solving certain types of problems or satisfying certain types of curiosities that students have.

Niching Your Teaching

When you specialize in solving certain problems or in exploring certain curiosities, you attract students who already have some motivation to solve that problem.

Attraction is easy when someone _already wants_ what you have to offer.

Imagine that a new student wants help with a certain problem. You appear in front of them, offering the solution. They will sign up for your class immediately, because you have the solution they've been looking for.

But your expert status doesn't just help in attracting new students. It helps you retain the students you've attracted. They will stick with you longer, because you are helping them with <u>exactly</u> what they want. That translates into trust and loyalty from new students – and it all starts even before they sign up.

The way to get this "specialization authority" is by defining your niche in Tai Chi and Qigong.

Niche may be a term you are not familiar with. The word *niche* (I pronounce this word "neesh," though some people say "nitch") is used in business and marketing.

Here's the business definition of a niche:

> *"A <u>specialized</u> segment of the market for a <u>particular</u> kind of product or service. Denoting or relating to products, services, or interests that appeal to a <u>small</u>, <u>specialized</u> section of the population."*

The key words in this definition are *specialized, particular,* and *small.* A niche is a small group in a much larger market. It is a group that has a particular interest in a certain kind of product or service.

Usually, the interest for a specialized product or service is driven by <u>one or both</u> of two key desires:

1. The members of the niche have a pressing problem they'd like solved.

2. The members of the niche have a curiosity that they need help to explore.

Either of these two characteristics will make the members of the niche more motivated, especially if they are having a difficult time finding help with their problems or curiosity.

Niche Examples Outside of Tai Chi and Qigong

Let's look at some examples of niches <u>outside</u> of Tai Chi and Qigong.

We'll start with a popular sport, such as golf.

You might think that *golfing* is a niche, since not everyone plays golf. But many different people participate in golf for many different reasons. It's hard to think of a "typical" golfer who would represent so many different types of people who play.

If you start to scratch the surface though, you'll find that within this diverse group of golfers, there are sub-groups.

One division is between recreational golfers, and those who are more serious about their game. Recreational golfers play for fun. For them, it's enough to be outdoors on the links, and they don't really care about improving their skills or dropping a few strokes from their score. But there are also golfers who are a bit more competitive. They want to improve their scores, and are more serious about upgrading their golfing skills. Not only do they play golf, but they also spend at least some time off the course thinking about their game and looking for ways to improve it.

Now let's say you were a golfing instructor. Which type of student do you think would be more motivated to join you for in-person coaching? The recreational golfer out just to have fun, or the more competitive golfer looking to improve her score?

Certainly the more competitive golfer would be an ideal student. This is especially true if you offered to teach them specific skills, such as *how to drive farther off the tee,* or *how to improve the mechanics of their swing.* A competitive golfer would be more motivated to join your coaching program, and more dedicated to following through on your instruction.

As another example, let's take a profession, such as *salesperson.* Like with golf, many people are in sales, at all different levels in their organizations or businesses. The job title of *salesperson* includes everyone from the front-line sales clerk at a retail establishment all the way up to the Vice-President of Sales at a multinational firm. It's difficult to think of a "typical" salesperson.

But again, if you scratch the surface, you realize there are sub-groups among these salespersons. For example, there are salespeople in medium-to-large size companies who are responsible for negotiating contracts with new customers. In their position, they pin down the details of the services the customer needs, how their company will provide those services, the costs involved, and the delivery dates. Once all of those details are agreed on, they work towards finalizing the contract and having the customer sign on the dotted line.

Many of these higher-level salespeople earn commissions on the contracts they close. So they are often motivated to improve their negotiation skills.

If you were a *sales trainer,* you couldn't ask for a more dedicated client for your training programs - especially if you offer courses on improving their negotiating skills and increasing their commissions.

As another example, how about people who *travel*? That's a large group of people. Some people travel for business. Some travel for pleasure. Some travel only within their country. Others are international travelers. Some people travel just once a year for the family vacation. Others travel many times a year, for many different reasons.

Of course, many of these people are budget travelers, while others prefer to *travel in style, sparing no expense.*

Let's say you ran a *five-star resort and hotel.* Which type of traveler do you think it would be easier to attract to your property? The budget traveler or the *in style* traveler? Where should you focus your marketing efforts?

As another example, how about food? Just about everyone in the world eats at some point. So *eating* certainly wouldn't be a niche. But people eat in many different ways for many different reasons. Some people eat for pleasure. Some eat for health. Some people eat special diets because of medical conditions or to lose weight. Some people eat meat, some people are vegetarians, and some people are vegans. Some people are gluttons, who'll eat anything. Some people are gourmets who are connoisseurs of good food.

But let's say you owned a *vegan* restaurant. If you tried to widely appeal to all of these types of eaters, you would struggle to find a regular clientele. But if you focused on the niche of *vegan eaters,* and provided them with healthy, delicious vegan offerings, you couldn't get a more dedicated group of restaurant goers for your business.

Just from these few examples, you can see that a niche contains people who have particular problems or interests.

And as you might imagine, people in niches are more *motivated* to find products or services that solve their problems and satisfy their interests than people who have only a mild curiosity about the subject.

Examples of Tai Chi and Qigong Niches

So how does this apply to your teaching?

In Tai Chi and Qigong, many instructors try to attract *anyone* to their classes and programs. They then try to motivate the *casually interested* students they find, in order to keep them coming back to their classes.

Sometimes this works, but it certainly is the hard way to do it. You'll wind up kissing a lot of frogs. And if you do happen to attract some frogs, you then have to work hard to motivate them into becoming princes and princesses.

Instead though, it would be far easier to skip over the frogs, and to look for "royalty" right from the start.

In other words, **start by looking for students who already have a special reason for learning Tai Chi or Qigong.**

As long as you can help them find what they are looking for, you'll find your classes full of Qi princes and princesses, not amphibians.

To do this, you can use the power of *niching* (pronounced "nee-shing" or "nitching") for your classes, workshops, and programs.

Start by looking for people:

- Who have a specific problem you can solve using Tai Chi or Qigong,

  … or …

- Who are curious about and looking for a specific "something" in Tai Chi or Qigong – but are having a hard time finding someone to explain it or show it to them.

The best way to think about this and get a feel for it is to look at some examples. So let me give you a few examples of qi-related niches.

As you read through these examples, pay attention to how each niche addresses a <u>particular group of people</u> who have a <u>particular problem</u> or a <u>particular curiosity</u>.

Here are eight examples of Tai Chi and Qigong niches:

1. Helping seniors with arthritis gain some relief from pain and increase their flexibility, making it easier to move in daily life.

2. Helping diabetic sufferers lower their blood sugar and lose weight.

3. Helping martial artists add "soft, internal energy" techniques to their self-defense skills.

4. Helping people use Tai Chi to improve their health, but who've been frustrated when other programs required them to memorize complex choreography or practice a lot each day.

5. Helping people actually experience and feel qi, especially if they've been disappointed by a lack of practical experience with other Tai Chi and Qigong classes.

6. Helping people with injuries caused by improper Tai Chi and Qigong to become aware of how to use their bodies properly to heal current problems and prevent any further damage.

7. Helping experienced students discover ways to overcome the physical, mental, and emotional roadblocks that prevent them from reaching higher-level qi skills and becoming masters.

8. Helping masters and teachers develop the client skills they need to attract and keep new students before they start teaching.

As you read through those examples, you may have noticed that they all address a particular type of person, and a particular problem or curiosity that that person would have.

In reading through these examples, I'm hoping you are starting to see and understand the power of niching.

Just imagine what will happen the next time you sign up new students. Visualize the difference between saying merely, "I teach Qigong," and saying more authoritatively "I help diabetic sufferers lower their blood sugar and lose weight with Qigong."

Or think about the difference between weakly saying "I teach Tai Chi," and expertly saying "I help people who want to experience and feel qi, even if they've been to other Tai Chi classes and never felt it before."

Focusing on certain problems or curiosities conveys almost instant authority and expert status – which translates to attracting motivated, dedicated students more easily.

By the way, I <u>don't</u> want you to think that the examples above were just part of some sort of "academic exercise" or "thought experiment." I also don't want you to think that these are all just "made up" examples.

While I did make up the first three examples, the last five are actually niches that I work in. The last five are some of <u>my niches</u> – the ones I teach in and create courses and programs for. They are real niches that I myself use.

Examples of "Non-Niches"

Now let's look at some counter-examples of teaching areas that are <u>not</u> niches.

I'm mentioning these here, because they are often the types of answers teachers give when prospective students asked, *"What do you teach?"*

But I think you'll see that these common answers are <u>not</u> niches. They <u>don't</u> address a particular group of people with a particular problem or curiosity.

From our perspective, these are "non-niches." Because of that, they don't convey the status or expert authority we need to attract new students.

As a matter of fact, it's even worse than that. These answers often leave prospective students with the impression that you are "just another teacher," interchangeable with many other run-of-the-mill Tai Chi and Qigong teachers.

Here are our first two "non-niche" answers:

- *"I teach Eight Brocades Qigong."*

- *"I teach Chen Style Tai Chi."*

When a new student asks *"what do you teach?"* it's common for teachers to answer with the styles and forms they teach. But these aren't niches. They don't identify the group of people the teaching is for, or the problem or curiosity being addressed. You may think that the style you teach is something special. But especially to a new prospect – someone who hasn't done Tai Chi or Qigong before – it doesn't make you special. It makes you "just another" Tai Chi or Qigong teacher.

Likewise ...

- *"I teach old Yang Style Tai Chi, as it was taught by founder Master Yang Lu-Chan."*

- *"I teach Wild Goose Qigong, and I am a lineage holder in the style."*

Some teachers answer the question "what do you teach" by mentioning their tradition, their lineage, or their certifications.

Credentials like these are important, but they are <u>not</u> niches. There's no mention of the type of person the teaching is aimed at, or the problems being solved or the curiosity being satisfied. There's nothing there to capture the interest of new students and motivate them to join your class.

Sometimes teachers will say ...

- *"I teach qigong for health."*

- *"I teach tai chi for martial arts and self-defense."*

These may be better answers than the first few above, but they are still <u>not</u> niches. Neither of these mentions the type of person to be taught. And while they do mention areas of interest, the areas are general, not particular.

This next answer is quite common from Tai Chi teachers:

- *"I teach tai chi as a complete art in all of its aspects."*

I think you can see that this is the exact <u>opposite</u> of a niche. Many teachers believe a statement like this shows their expertise. And maybe it does to some students. But to a new student, it makes the teacher seem like a "jack of all trades," rather than someone who can help him with his specific expectations.

Finally, you sometimes hear these answers:

- *"I teach qigong for seniors."*

- *"I teach tai chi for arthritis."*

Those answers are slightly better than the others, but still much too general. "Seniors" or "people with arthritis" are groups that are much too large to be niches. You'd need to narrow them down to a particular problem that seniors or those with arthritis have in order to have a niche.

The whole goal of niching your teaching is that you want to attract motivated, dedicated students. So you want your answer to the question *"what do you teach?"* to create a certain response in the prospective students.

When you tell a new student what you teach, you want him to respond with *"Hey, that's me! This teacher knows exactly what I want. This might be the right teacher for me!"*

So by focusing on a particular niche – that is a group of people who have a specific problem or specific curiosity – you give yourself the maximum power to attract loyal, committed students.

Objecting to Niching

I realize this idea of niching probably makes sense to you in the abstract, or at least in these specific examples.

But when we start talking about your classes, your programs, your students, and your promotions, that's usually where this gets difficult.

Most Qi teachers are afraid to niche their teaching.

They already have trouble finding students, so they are afraid that by "limiting" themselves to certain niches, they'll have an even harder time finding students.

So instead, they try to appeal broadly to anyone who might be interested in Tai Chi or Qigong. They figure that the more broadly they appeal, the easier it will be to find students.

After all, with all of the competition they have for students, how could they afford to turn away anyone who might be interested in their classes?

But in reality, appealing broadly like this is exactly why finding new students is a problem for them.

First of all, appealing broadly makes them *vulnerable to the competition*. It turns the teacher into a "little fish in a big pond" that is full of fish all competing against each other.

It means they are competing for the exact same students that every other teacher of Tai Chi or Qigong is competing for - and they are competing for them in the exact same way every other teacher does.

When they appeal broadly to students, they don't give new students any special reason to study with them. The students might just as easily choose any other teacher.

After all, all of these "broadly appealing" teachers start to look the same to new students. They may think, *"Tai Chi is Tai Chi, isn't it? So what does it matter what class I join?"*

Appealing broadly to people actually creates that reaction in prospective students. In their minds, your class becomes interchangeable with every other Tai Chi or Qigong class.

The result of this? You no longer "stand out," and you lose any expert status, authority, and credibility you might have had.

Besides making the teacher vulnerable to competition, "not specializing" is also why retention rates for new students are generally low.

When teachers cast a wide net like that, they wind up with a lot of *mildly interested - but not necessarily motivated* – students. These are the students that lose interest and quit easily.

They also wind up with students who have widely different expectations – most of which the class and the teacher will fail to meet.

Finally, the students they do attract are also the ones more susceptible to being lured away by the competition - such as other teachers, other programs, online courses, video, and even the inertia we talked about earlier.

Now, it's true that taking a niche approach actually will <u>drive away</u> some prospective students. But usually they are the ones who are only mildly curious or who lack motivation. They are the ones that are <u>least likely</u> to stick around.

On the other hand, when you specialize in solving certain problems or in exploring certain curiosities, you attract students who <u>already</u> are motivated to learn from you and stick with you.

They want their problem solved, or their curiosity explored. You are offering to help them do that. Imagine how motivating that would be to a prospective student.

Presenting yourself as an expert in a specialized area makes it easier to attract and retain students who feel like you are addressing exactly what they want. You gain a lot of authority – which translates into trust and loyalty from new students.

They feel like you are speaking directly to them, in a way that other teachers don't.

So the solution to most student attraction and retention problems is to niche.

As marketer Dan Kennedy once described niching, you don't want to swim in a big ocean with everyone else. Instead, you want to find a small puddle and jump up and down on top of it, splashing as much as you can.

That puddle, where you can make a big splash, is your niche.

The Power of Niche Intersection

For Tai Chi and Qigong teachers, there are two major ways to find a niche for your teaching:

1. You can look at problems <u>you</u> want to solve or maybe that you have already solved for yourself and others. You can also look at areas <u>you</u> are curious about and would like to explore.

2. You can look at problems <u>others</u> want to solve or that <u>others</u> are curious about.

So you could find a niche that's about what <u>you</u> want or a niche that's about what <u>others</u> want.

Now, you could choose just one of these ways to find a niche. But I wouldn't recommend it. Doing just one or the other has problems.

For example, you could choose a niche that you are interested in. But you might find that others <u>aren't</u> interested in that niche. So you may have trouble attracting students if there aren't many others around that are also interested.

On the other hand, you could choose niches others want, even if you have <u>no</u> interest in the niche yourself. But if you do that, you might find yourself losing motivation for teaching. Teaching can become boring and tedious, almost soulless, if you yourself aren't really interested in what you are teaching.

So you can do one or the other, but doing an *intersection* of both gives you the best *attraction power* possible.

Finding problems you <u>and</u> others are interested in makes this whole process work more smoothly.

Now when choosing niches, you may have to consider your *reach* – the locations where you teach and the students that are available in those locations. Your reach may limit what niches you have available to you. We'll talk more about this in our upcoming chapter on teaching locations.

But for now, the best "bang for your buck" is to look at the niches where both you <u>and</u> others have a compelling interest.

The Two List Method for Finding Niches

Here's a method you can use to find your *niche intersection*.

I'd like you to create two lists.

The first is a list of problems you want to solve or areas you are curious about. The second is a list of problems others want to solve or areas others are curious about

Let start with the first list. List #1 is all about you. List out all of the special interests you have in Tai Chi and Qigong. This could be problems you've solved for yourself or curiosities you have. It could be skills you are already expert in, or that you'd like to become expert in. It could be subjects or skills that you've already taught and enjoyed teaching, or it could even be topics you don't know about, but would like to learn about for yourself and to teach to others.

Any sub-topic in Tai Chi or Qigong that captures your interest should be on List #1.

Moving on to List #2, this list is all about others. List the types of problems that others have an interest in solving or subjects they are curious about.

So how do you build List #2?

If you are already in a class – either as a teacher or as a student - start by asking the other students in the class about their problems or curiosities in Tai Chi and Qigong.

If you are the teacher of the class, you can just start a class discussion on the topic.

If you are a student in the class, you can just casually ask other members of the class either before or after class, or during break times in the class. Most people love to talk about their interests and their problems, so it's not hard to get them to open up about why they want to learn Tai Chi or Qigong.

Also, if you are a student, you may want to ask your teachers about their interests. Why do they like Tai Chi or Qigong, and what are they most interested in? Teachers like to talk about themselves just like everyone else. Plus, since most teachers don't niche, they may actually have niches they are interested in but have never talked about.

For List #2, you might also want to look around your "community" – whether that's your local city, your national or international connections, or your online connections. Check with people you know to see what problems they are worrying about, or what curiosities they may have, that you might be able to satisfy with Tai Chi or Qigong. Also check the media and gathering places (online and offline) to see what problems others are talking about. You might also want to check relevant publications and professional organizations for ideas.

Also check out the competition – other teachers in your area – to find the "holes" in niches in your area. See what niches other Qi teachers may be missing in their promotions in order to see if you can provide what they aren't providing. You can do this easily with some online searches for websites and announcements for classes and programs from other teachers.

Speaking of being online, you can also do web searches for *"tai chi forums"* or *"qigong forums."* Read the posts on these forums that have the <u>largest number of responses</u>. The more responses to a forum post, the more likely that post hits a niche where people are in need of help.

Also, do a similar search on social media, searching for *"tai chi"* or *"qigong."* Find the accounts and pages that have the most interaction to see what others are talking about.

If you are more adept with online tools, you can look at *"search trends"* online. Most search engines have a place where you can find the most popular searches in Tai Chi and Qigong. The search counts can help you find niches that others are searching for.

Here's one important note about creating List #2. **This list should be about niches people <u>want</u>, not what they <u>need</u>.**

You may find a group of people who could really use help with a problem, but they <u>don't recognize</u> that they have the problem. Or maybe they know they have a problem, but they've <u>not</u> expressed that they even want help with it.

If that's the case, it's usually <u>not</u> a good niche.

It can be a frustrating experience trying to convince people not just that you can help them, but that they even need help in the first place. So as you do this niche research for List #2, **focus on what people actually say they <u>want</u>, not on what you might think they need.**

Using the Two Lists

Once you have both lists, look at them, and see if you can find any topics in common between the two.

If you find a topic that is on both lists, you've found an ideal niche for yourself.

When both you <u>and</u> others are interested in the same subject, you've found an extremely satisfying and potentially successful niche to build your courses and programs around.

Now, that sometimes happens, but more often, you'll find that there are topics that aren't completely common, but somewhat related between the two lists. They may not be identical, but they are really close. If so, those would be good niches.

Of course, you might find that there is nothing at all in common between your two lists. That does happen sometimes. In that case, I suggest looking at List #2 (the "others" list), and seeing if there's a topic there you hadn't thought of for yourself, but that you'd actually be curious about. That would make a good niche.

If you can't find anything like that, you might have to consider expanding your *reach*. You may have to expand the types of locations you are looking at, or the types of people you are looking at, and create a new List #2 for those people.

For example, if you are a local teacher, and you made List #2 based mostly on what your current students tell you, you may have to look outside of your students. You may have to check your local community for a wider selection for List #2.

After all of this though, it's still possible that you can't find a niche on List #2 that you want. In that case, just choose something from List #1, your own list. Keep in mind that you'll have a harder time attracting students if it's a niche you want and others don't want. You may have to look long and hard to find new students that fit your particular wants.

Crafting Your Niche Statements

In the end though, you should come up with two to five niches you could teach from these two lists. Once you've done that, take the possible niches you've found, and create a good "niche statement" for each of them.

A niche statement is a single sentence that describes the niche. Your niche statements should focus on the people and on their specific problems or on the specific curiosities they have.

To help you craft your niche statements, let's use the eight examples of Tai Chi and Qigong niches we listed earlier in this chapter. You can use these examples as *models* for your own niche statements.

Let me repeat those eight examples here for you. Notice how each example starts with the word "helping," followed by the group of people being helped, and then followed by the exact problem we're solving or curiosity we're exploring.

1. Helping seniors with arthritis gain some relief from pain and increase their flexibility, making it easier to move in daily life.

2. Helping diabetic sufferers lower their blood sugar and lose weight.

3. Helping martial artists add "soft, internal energy" techniques to their self-defense skills.

4. Helping people use Tai Chi to improve their health, but who've been frustrated when other programs required them to memorize complex choreography or practice a lot each day.

5. Helping people actually experience and feel qi, especially if they've been disappointed by a lack of

practical experience with other Tai Chi and Qigong classes.

6. Helping people with injuries caused by improper Tai Chi and Qigong to become aware of how to use their bodies properly, to help heal current problems and prevent any further damage.

7. Helping experienced students discover ways to overcome the physical, mental, and emotional roadblocks that prevent them from reaching higher-level qi skills.

8. Helping teachers develop the skills they need to attract and keep new students before they start teaching.

When you write your own niche statements, follow the same model used in these examples. That model is:

Helping [a particular group of people] to [do something] for [their particular problem or curiosity].

Using this model, take the two to five niches you found on your niche lists, and write niche statements for each one.

Once you have your new niche statements in hand, you'll be ready to take the next step – identifying your ideal students in each niche. We'll get to that in the next chapter.

Action Items

Note: At the end of most chapters, you'll find one or more *action items*. To get the most out of your new "student attraction" approach to teaching, make sure you **complete these action items before moving on to the next chapter.**

Find My Teaching Niches

- Create two lists:

    1. Problems and areas I'm curious about.

    2. Problems others want solved

- Find topics in common in both lists.

- No common topics found? Look on #2 for topics I'd like to explore.

- Still none? Expand my reach to create a new #2 list to look for new topics.

- Still none? Pick topics from #1 list.

- Goal: Find two to five niches from these lists.

- Create a niche statement for each of these niches in this format: "Helping [a particular group of people] to [do something] for [their particular problem or curiosity]."

Identifying Your Ideal Students

Kristen is in her late 40's or early 50's. It's hard to tell though, because she likes to take care of herself. She's very much into health.

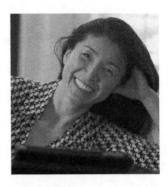

For example, since she works only part-time (she and her husband do well financially), she has the time to prepare organic and healthy meals for herself, her husband, and her two teenagers.

She's <u>not</u> an avid exerciser, but not too long ago, she took a few Tai Chi classes. She enjoyed the classes, but with family and part-time work, she didn't have as much time to practice outside of class as she would like. But she'd take classes again if they fit her schedule and were near where she lives.

Howard has been reading a lot about Tai Chi and Qigong lately.

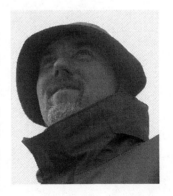

He studied martial arts when he was in grade school, but that was a long time ago. He was thinking about getting started again, but then he came across some articles online about "qi." He'd really like to know more about this "life energy."

But he doesn't really know where to start. He's looked at a few videos and books, and while there's a lot of talk about qi, the videos don't seem to live up to the hype. A lot of it seems like the karate he learned in his youth, just done more slowly. He doesn't really see the connection between the movements and this "life energy" stuff. That's what he'd like to know about.

Howard does well at his job, so he has both time and funds to spend to learn. He just doesn't know where to start.

Mary has been studying Tai Chi for many years, and she's even done some teaching herself. She's a dedicated practitioner. She's frequently travelled to workshops around the country. To her, it's more than a hobby. It's an integral part of her life and her identity.

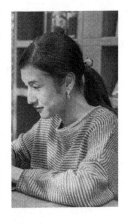

But she's recently noticed some knee pain from her practice. It's not a lot of pain, and doesn't bother her much, but it seems to happen only after she does her Tai Chi forms.

At first, she didn't connect it with her practice, especially since she knows that Tai Chi does so many great things for health. She thought it might be old age catching up with her.

But then she noticed that the pain always happens <u>after</u> practice. What concerns her is that the pain is starting to linger a little longer after each session.

Peter, to put it bluntly, wants to be a master.

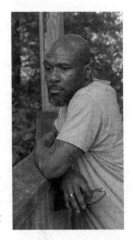

He's had decades of experience learning and teaching Qigong and Tai Chi, but he always feels like something is holding him back a bit. He sees other masters he admires, and he feels like he could be one of them, with all of his experience. But he feels like he's still missing something. He's just not certain what that something is.

Peter also tends to be a bit of a loner, which he thinks holds him back a bit. While he likes going to classes and workshops, he feels like the "real work" in Tai Chi and Qigong is done on your own. But he feels like he's stuck at the "advanced student" level, and really wants to breakthrough to the next level - whatever that might be.

Student Avatars

Depending on your teaching niche in Tai Chi and Qigong, *Kristen, Howard, Mary,* and *Peter* sound like they could be perfect students. And indeed they are perfect – maybe a little too perfect - because they aren't real.

Kristen, Howard, Mary, and Peter are imaginary "ideal students" – ones I created for various courses and projects I've done in Tai Chi and Qigong.

In the marketing world, these imaginary, ideal people are called *customer avatars* – fictional characters that represent the "model prospects" in a given niche.

However, for Qigong and Tai Chi, we can think of these profiles as *student avatars,* or just simply as your *ideal students.*

Niching Down Even More

We talked about niches in the last chapter – those groups of people who have a certain problem or a certain curiosity that you can help with Tai Chi and Qigong.

But there are lots of people in any niche. Some you can help, and some you can't, for various reasons.

So putting together an "ideal student" profile helps you narrow down the niche even more – to the exact type of students in the niche you want to work with.

Having an ideal student in mind helps you attract the right students to your class, workshop, or program. It helps you craft your offers and communication to address the types of students you work best with.

When you are just starting to put together a new course or program, it's difficult to wrap your mind around a group of individuals.

It's much easier to craft your message if you are talking to <u>an individual</u>, even if they are imaginary.

Imagining a person, rather than a group, gives you greater insight into who your prospective students are and what they want.

Ironically, an *imaginary* student is a way to make *more real* your own desires as far as the type of student you want to attract.

Especially at the beginning stages – when you are first thinking of teaching a new course and first putting together a promotion for it – an ideal student profile keeps you focused on the important question: *"Who is this for?"*

Having an ideal student in mind from the beginning makes it more likely that your message will attract the prospective students who are right for you, your class, your teaching method, and your subject.

They will sign up, even if they don't *exactly* fit the ideal profile.

Of course, the majority of your students <u>won't</u> exactly fit the ideal.

Some may have a few characteristics in common with the ideal, but rarely will a new student fit it exactly. But usually your new students are *responding* to the ideal – that is, something about the ideal will be attractive to them. That's why they'll sign up, and also what will motivate them to keep coming back for more.

And often, the wrong students – the ones that <u>don't</u> fit what you teach or how you teach, and will most likely be dissatisfied and quit – will be <u>turned off</u> by the ideal student profile. It will stop them from joining your class in the first place.

Just imagine what this does <u>positively</u> to your retention rate - not to mention to your own motivation and enthusiasm - when you don't have to deal with students that aren't right for you and what you teach.

That's the power of these ideal student avatars.

The Power of Student Avatars

This whole idea of "avatars" is another skill I learned the hard way. As I mentioned earlier, when I started teaching, I had no background in business or marketing. So it was only later that I found out that avatars were a "thing" used in business.

My first attempts weren't really avatars though. They were just "lists" of characteristics of some of my students.

You'll soon see though how even these crude lists caused me to see a major flaw in my approach to teaching. (More about that in the next chapter.)

But once I eventually learned about "avatars," it made my student attraction all that much more effective. It made it easier for me to conceive of, promote, and even teach new classes, workshops, and programs to both my new and existing students.

Today, I don't do a single project without having an avatar in mind.

I have an avatar in mind for each niche, and for each course or program I develop for that niche.

I sometimes even have a different avatar for each "lesson" or "module" in a course.

For example, many of you have been in my programs where I provide you with something monthly – like a newsletter, a monthly video, or a monthly audio. I always have an avatar in mind before I create that monthly training.

This even extends down to when I send out emails. Some of you have been on my email lists and gotten daily or weekly emails from me. <u>Every single one</u> of those emails was written with an avatar in mind.

Developing Your Avatars

So how do you develop your avatars?

One of the greatest sources of avatars is *students you already have.*

I mentioned that I always have an avatar in mind when I write my newsletters or do my videos and audios.

Well, many times, those avatars based on actual students who have asked me questions that led to the creation of the training. So I keep the actual person in mind as my avatar when I create the training.

Another great source of avatars is *students you've observed* when you've been in another teacher's class or program.

Many times, I've been at a workshop, and I've seen a fellow student who asks a question or makes a comment. His remarks might lead me to think about a niche I hadn't thought of. I may even later create a course or program for the niche. Well, as I explore the niche, I keep him in mind as my avatar for the niche.

People you meet outside of classes can be a source of avatars. Sometimes, a person will say or do something that leads you to realize they have a problem or curiosity that Tai Chi or Qigong could solve. In other words, you've found someone who is a member of a *niche,* even if she doesn't know it herself. So you realize that she might make a great avatar for certain niches you explore.

This is also true with people you see online, in forums and on social media, especially as you are doing the niche research we described in the last chapter.

Also, don't forget your own imagination. You can imagine who your ideal student would be, and use that imaginary ideal student as a source for your avatar's characteristics.

Finally you can create avatars by thinking about difficult students you've had in the past. If you don't like or work well with particular types of students, you can use them as *negative examples* – that is, as the types of students who should not be your avatar. Use these negative examples to create a positive avatar who has different or opposite characteristics to these problem students.

But usually, your ideal student won't be from just one source. Usually, your avatar will be a composite made from some or all of these sources.

For example, you may take some characteristics from a student you have, plus some parts from someone who asked a question in an online forum, plus a bit of your imagination. You might put all of that together to make your ideal student.

Your Avatar's Details

In business and marketing, these avatars are usually highly detailed. If you've ever seen a company's ideal customer profile, it may go into great detail on this imaginary person's life.

They'll not only name the person, they'll name the person's spouse and children. They'll talk about where they live and work. They'll talk about their job and coworkers, sometimes even naming the coworkers. They'll mention the stores their avatar shops at, the restaurants they eat at, and the cars they drive. They'll talk about their hobbies and interests, the websites they visit, the books they read, and the television shows they watch. These avatar profiles can be highly detailed, and run for pages and pages of text.

Thankfully, our avatars <u>don't</u> need to be this detailed.

My first attempts at avatars were crude. Mostly they were just lists of characteristics. That's how I got started with avatars.

But now, my avatars are much like the ones from the start of this chapter.

I write two or three paragraphs that tell the basic story and characteristics of the avatar, as it relates to the niche I'm working in, and the problems I'm solving for that niche.

These days, I work in some well-defined niches, and now I mostly teach only masters, teachers, and students I already know or who have been in my previous classes and programs. So quite often, my avatars are real people.

(Maybe even <u>you</u> have been one of my avatars before. You might even be the avatar I used to create this book!)

Since I know my avatars well, it's easy to write a few paragraphs about them.

You may have noticed that along with the few paragraphs I wrote for the avatars at the start of this chapter, I also included photos.

Of course, these photos <u>aren't really</u> Kristen, Howard, Mary, and Peter, because those four people don't exist. Instead, the photos are just model photos I found on a photo-sharing website that gave me a license to use these photos for this book.

When I create my avatars, I don't usually include photos like I did here. I did that just as an example for you.

But many people swear by having a photo to associate with their avatar. It makes the avatar more "real" to them.

If having a photo would help you, by all means, use one.

You can go online to social media and photo-sharing websites to find photos that you think best depicts your avatar – even if the person in the photo might not actually be an ideal student.

Note: If you do use web photos, I do want to caution you about copyright issues. As the law stands in the U.S. at the time that I'm writing this, you can use a photo on the web for your <u>private use</u> as an avatar. That is, as long as you won't be sharing the photo with others or publishing your student profiles anywhere, you can use any online photo as an avatar.

Of course, I rarely publish my avatar profiles. This book is an exception. You probably won't share your profiles either. So since your profiles and photos will be for your own use, you won't need a license for them.

But if you are publishing your avatar profiles or making them available for public consumption, you'll need a license to use the photo. Do not publish other people's photos without the appropriate license and permission.

Reminder: I'm not a lawyer. So you should consult legal counsel for the laws in your area before taking any advice from this book.

As I said, I usually don't use photos. I did though include the photos (which I licensed) at the beginning of this chapter as examples.

But whether you use a photo or not, your avatar <u>doesn't</u> need a lot of detail. You just need to include enough details to make them "real" for you and to help you focus.

Using Your Student Avatars

Your "ideal student" helps with promoting your courses.

When you write your course descriptions, your ads, your flyers – whatever media you use to get new students – you write to that ideal student. When you put together your class and organize your teaching material, keep that ideal student in mind. If you use a photo, have the photo in front of you as you do your work.

The first night of class, you'll be talking to and about your ideal student, especially when you first introduce yourself, and introduce your class to your new students.

Of course, over time, as you get to know your new students, you'll talk more directly to them and to their needs.

But at the start, talking to and about your ideal student will help connect you to these students who already are *attracted to* and responded to the ideal student you used to create the course.

Those are all important reasons for having a student profile. But your ideal student profile is even more important for the next step in our Zero Drop Outs Strategy – finding out where your ideal students are.

Creating Your Avatars

Before we get to that next step though, you'll need to get some practice in creating student avatars.

To do this, just take the niches you identified in the last chapter, and create an ideal student profile for each niche.

Write out two or three paragraphs that describe your ideal student in each niche.

You can base this on students you've had before, on people you found doing niche research, or on people you come up with using your imagination.

Give your ideal students names to help make them more real. If you'd like, look on social media or on photo-sharing websites for a photo for each ideal student.

If you need help with writing your profiles, you can use the profiles for Kristen, Howard, Mary, and Peter that I gave at the start of this chapter as models.

Don't worry about making these ideal student profiles perfect. Just do this as an exercise to get in the habit of thinking about your ideal students, and to get some practice with creating student avatars.

We'll use your student avatars in the next chapter.

Action Items

Identify My Ideal Students

For each niche on my list from the previous step:

- Write two or three paragraphs describing my ideal student avatar in that niche.

- *Give each avatar a name, and describe any general characteristics (age, gender, income, education, family, hobbies, interests, etc.).*
- *Specifically focus on the avatar's interest in Tai Chi or Qigong, and what problems they want solved or curiosities they have.*
- *Optional: Look on social media or on photo-sharing websites for a photo for the avatar. (Photos should be for your private use only.)*
- *Don't worry about getting these avatars perfect - just get them done!*

Finding Where Your Ideal Students Are

During my first eight years of teaching, I taught at three different types of facilities.

I taught at two different health centers, attached to a local hospital and insurance company. I also taught at a facility run by a city parks and recreation department. Finally, I taught at two different locations in the same corporate business park.

All but one of these were convenient locations for me. They were all around Hillsboro, Oregon, where I lived and worked (back when I had a "day" job).

During those years, I had somewhere around 500 to 700 people per year join my beginning classes. If that number seems high, keep in mind that most of those people joined at the health centers, having been referred by the hospital and insurance company.

But after eight years of having 500 to 700 beginners, I had only around fifteen to twenty students that stuck with me for two years or longer.

That started to bother me.

Out of that many beginners, why did 96% or more quit within two years?

What was I doing wrong?

89

I thought a lot about those who quit. Often times, I would have someone I considered to be a promising student quit just after a few classes.

Why did that happen?

My First Student Profile

After a while, I realized I was focusing on the wrong side of this here.

I shouldn't spend time wondering about the quitters.

Instead, I should focus my attention on those who <u>stayed</u>.

One day, I sat down and thought about my long-term students. The fifteen to twenty who stayed long-term were certainly a motley crew – different ages, different genders, and different occupations. When it came to Tai Chi and Qigong, they had different interests, different skill levels, and different experience levels.

At first glance, it seemed like these individuals had nothing in common. But the more I thought about them, I realized they did have a few things in common.

I made a list of their common characteristics:

- Most of these students were interested in health. They were already in fairly good health, or maybe had some minor problems. But they wanted to be more healthy overall, and had a general interest in health, including exercise, nutrition, and lifestyle.

- Most of these long-term students either didn't have children, or had children that were older teenagers or that no longer lived at home. So they had time in their life for classes. A few exceptions had younger children, but they also had one spouse who could take care of the children while the other parent attended classes.

- Most had work or family schedules that allowed them at least some time – say 10 to 20 minutes each day - for practice.

- Most were either white collar workers, stay-at-home parents, or part-time workers in their family. Most came from households that had disposable income to afford classes.

- Nearly all of my long-term students had been to other Tai Chi or Qigong classes, or in some cases yoga classes, before coming to my class. They could recognize and value that what we offered in our classes was different from more "standard" approaches to Tai Chi and Qigong.

- Many were already interested in qi in some fashion either before or shortly after they joined the class.

That list was my first crude "student avatar" – though I hadn't heard that term at that time.

But something struck me about the people on this list versus the other students at the health centers, the parks department, and the business park.

At the hospital health centers, most of the students who registered had <u>never been</u> to another Tai Chi or Qigong class before. Some <u>hadn't even seen</u> Tai Chi before and knew nothing about it when they signed up.

Most were there because they were told Tai Chi would be good for them or their health problems. But I'd have to say that most <u>had never been committed to health</u> before in their lives, which in some cases had led to their health problems in the first place. In most cases, they were there because they felt like they <u>had to be</u> because of their problems, not because they wanted to be there. They "needed" to improve their health, but they didn't necessarily "want" Tai Chi or Qigong.

Finally, most of these health centers students didn't have to pay for classes. Their insurance company paid for them. So they had no financial stake in their participation.

The students at the city parks and recreations department mostly came from blue-collar and lower middle class living situations without much disposable income. Like at the hospital, most of the students <u>had never been</u> to another Tai Chi or Qigong class before.

Most were only <u>mildly interested</u> in exercise. Several said they had originally intended to sign up for a different class, but my course description caught their attention. Some had children that attended the same facility for day-care – that's how they found my class.

Finally, the classes at this location were low-cost, subsidized by the city. Again, the students had little financial incentive to attend and succeed

At the corporate business park where I taught, I had a different type of student. Most were high-tech workers who were <u>not</u> that interested in health. But like the other locations, most had never seen Tai Chi or Qigong before.

A number of them were past and present coworkers of mine. They knew I taught Tai Chi, and they were just curious about it. Sometimes we had "outsiders" - those who didn't work in the business park - attend classes. But they tended <u>not</u> to stick around, because the commute to that area was difficult during rush hour.

Finding the Right Location

Notice that the short-term students at these three locations did <u>not</u> fit the profile of my long-term students.

While my long-term students came from these locations, they were the *exceptions* to the majority of students who signed up at the health centers, the parks and rec center, and the business park.

So comparing the list of characteristics of my long term students – that is, my first crude student avatar – to the types of students who came to these locations led me to a realization.

And it may just have been the single biggest realization that led me to become the successful teacher I eventually became.

That realization was that ...

I was teaching at the wrong locations.

I was teaching at places that <u>didn't attract</u> the types of students I worked best with, that I enjoyed teaching, and that often became my long-term students..

So why was I teaching at these places?

I made a classic mistake that a lot of teachers make. I was teaching at places that were convenient to me, in terms of locations and availability.

Though they were convenient, these locations were in areas of the city and in facilities that were <u>not</u> likely to pull in the students that I worked best with. It's like I was fishing at the wrong lakes with the wrong bait.

I realize that I either had to change <u>what</u> I was using for bait, or change <u>where</u> I was fishing. That is, I either had to change <u>what</u> I was teaching or <u>where</u> I was teaching if I wanted to be successful.

Well, I enjoyed <u>what</u> I was teaching, and I enjoyed working with my current long term students. I realized I'd rather teach more students who were like them.

So I kept the bait, but went looking for new fishing holes.

The Criteria

Though I lived in Hillsboro, Oregon, I was fortunate in the fact that I was close to the larger city of Portland, Oregon. This city had lots of different suburbs, communities, and smaller cities around it.

So I went looking for an area of Portland and a facility that was likely to attract what my long-term student profile showed me.

In other words, I wanted to find a place that had:

- Students from primarily white-collar households with disposable income.

- Students for whom child care was not a problem.

- Students that had schedules that allowed for a weekly class plus 10-20 minutes a day to practice.

- Students who were interested in a healthy lifestyle.

- Students who had been to "alternative exercise" classes before (Tai Chi, Qigong, Yoga, Pilates, etc.).

- Students who were already interested or could become interested in *qi* in some fashion.

Well, I found a location.

Of course, this location was <u>not</u> convenient like the others I had been teaching at. During rush hour, when I would leave my day job to go teach, it could be up to an hour drive to get there. The return drive after class, at night when the roads were clear, could be a half-hour to forty-five minutes. So I would spend almost two hours in the car getting there and back.

But even though the new location wasn't convenient to me, **it was convenient in the one way that counted. It was where my students were,** so it made it easy to find the new students I wanted.

Checking the Demographics

The new location was in Lake Oswego, Oregon, a small city near Portland.

The demographics, as shown in the chart below, were much more in line with my long-term students. That's especially true when compared to the demographics of Hillsboro, where I had been teaching.

	Hillsboro, OR	Lake Oswego, OR
Population	71,000	35,000
Prior decade growth	80%	15%
Age	23% over age 45	42% over age 45
Per capita income	$22,000	$42,000

Median income	$57,000	$72,000
Households with children	9,530	4,700
Teaching Location	Hospital centers, parks department, corporate business park	Fitness center inside a natural foods store

This chart goes back a few years, back when I moved my classes, so the demographics are different today.

But at the time, the population of Hillsboro where I was teaching was 71,000 people, where Lake Oswego had a population of less than half that amount. Lake Oswego was a much smaller community.

In the prior decade, Hillsboro had grown by 80%, whereas Lake Oswego had only grown 15%. So the smaller size with less growth meant that Lake Oswego had an older, longer established, and more stable population.

The age differences between the two cities were dramatic. Hillsboro had a younger population, with only 23% of its citizens over the age of 45. Lake Oswego, percentage-wise, had almost double the amount of older adults. Since I was looking for students for whom child care was not a problem, an older population generally worked better.

The per capita and median incomes also contributed here. Lake Oswego had nearly double the per capita income of Hillsboro. The median income in Lake Oswego was 25% higher.

Both of those figures meant Lake Oswego had a primarily white collar population with more disposable income. Generally, white collar households with disposable income often (though not always) means the prospective students have space in their schedules for classes and for daily practice. So this all fit better with the long-term profile of the students I was already attracting.

Finally, in Hillsboro, over 9,500 households had children, while only 4,700 had children in Lake Oswego. Now that's relatively in proportion in both populations But considering that Hillsboro had mostly younger adults, most of those children in Hillsboro were younger too. Child care was a potential problem for parents wanting to take classes. Lake Oswego with its older population had fewer younger children that would require child care.

Finding the Right Facility

So putting this all together, you can see how Lake Oswego, despite a smaller population than Hillsboro, might make it easier for me to reach people who could potentially become long-term students.

The demographics in Lake Oswego fit for:

- Students from primarily white-collar households with disposable income.

- Students for whom child care was not a problem.

- Students that had schedules that allowed for a weekly class plus 10-20 minutes a day to practice.

But there were additional characteristics I was looking for. These included:

- Students who were interested in a healthy lifestyle.

- Students who had been to "alternative exercise" classes before (Tai Chi, Qigong, Yoga, Pilates, etc.).

- Students who were already interested or became interested in "qi" in some fashion.

So now that I had the right city, I had to find a facility in that city that fit with these characteristics.

In driving around Lake Oswego, I found the perfect teaching facility. I found a fitness center that was inside a natural foods store.

As you might imagine, people that are visiting a natural foods store are usually predisposed to one of my avatar characteristics - a healthy lifestyle. A fitness center inside a natural food store narrowed that down even farther to people with a healthy lifestyle that wanted to exercise.

At that fitness center, they were also already offering yoga classes, Pilates, and a few other alternative exercise classes. I believe they may have also had Tai Chi classes there at one time, but there were none currently.

(Even if there had been existing Tai Chi or Qigong classes, that wouldn't have deterred me. In the next chapter, when we talk about *class offerings,* you'll see competition isn't a problem even if your location already offers Tai Chi or Qigong classes from other instructors.)

But whether or not they had Tai Chi classes, there was already a pool of people attending similar classes at this location. This meant that this center attracted students who had some exposure to alternative exercises, another of my characteristics.

Of course, the final characteristic in my avatar list was "interest in qi." That one was hard to quantify from the demographics and the location. I had no idea at the time on how to find that. But the location had so many of the other characteristics that I decided not to worry about it.

The Power of the Right Location

As you might guess, holding courses in this city at that location made a significant difference in the types of students I could attract.

So if you add "right location" to the combination of "right niche" and "right student" – well, all three made it easy to fill my classes at that fitness center, and to keep them full.

I started by just teaching two classes on one night. But because of the number of students I was attracting, I was quickly able to expand my teaching schedule. I also started offering one-off workshops and a monthly workshop series, in addition to the ongoing classes. Getting enough students for all of these offerings was <u>no</u> problem. My classes started full, and they stayed full.

My drop-out immediately plummeted to fewer than 10% for the weekly classes, and eventually reached 0% for the last few years there. I stopped accepting new students for the final year, since all of my students were returning for each session. I had all the students I could handle.

When I finally stopped teaching the weekly classes, all of my students had been with me at least a year, most for several years.

The Role of Location

This experience is an example of the importance of "location" for a local teacher (me), teaching in-person classes, near a big city.

But location isn't just about physically where you teach.

It's also about "reach" – being able to find and connect with prospective students, wherever they are, to get them to your classes, workshops, or programs.

Reach can involve more than just a simple geographic location, especially if you teach something other than local classes.

If you teach national or international workshops, or if you teach through remote learning (online programs, video, books, etc.), reach can involve a lot more.

But let's talk a little more about geographic location first, before we move onto these other areas.

Discovering Your Attraction Priorities

So far, we've covered the first three steps of our Zero Drop Outs Strategy. These steps are: (1) Find your teaching niches, (2) Identify your ideal students, and (3) Find out where those students are.

We've talked about these three separately, and in a certain order. But these three steps actually influence each other, and should be considered together.

There's a priority to the first three steps of the Zero Drop Outs Strategy, and that priority depends on <u>you</u> and <u>your goals</u> in teaching.

It comes down to <u>why</u> you are a teacher.

For example, let's say you want to be an in-person, local teacher. You have no interest in travelling, or in becoming a national or international teacher. Your primary goal is to teach in your local community.

If that's the case, *location* is your teaching priority. So that should be the primary factor in your student attraction strategy.

As a result, depending on <u>where</u> you want to teach, you may find that your *ideal teaching niches* and *ideal students* are <u>not</u> available in your location.

For example, you may like teaching Tai Chi to martial artists, but you live in a small town of mostly retirees in a remote area. It is unlikely in that location you'll find enough martial artists in your niche. So you may have to change your niche and student avatar to match the people available in your location – once again, if location is your priority.

But let's say your *martial arts* niche and ideal students have priority over staying local. In that case, you may have to get out of your local area.

For example, you might want to become a national or international teacher to reach your prospective students. You could do this by travelling to teach workshops in areas where there are more martial artists. Or you might offer remote learning (books, videos, online) to martial artists around the country, and around the world. You would do that if your niche or your ideal student is a higher priority than your location.

Choosing Your Priority

It all comes down to the priorities that would satisfy you as a teacher. You have to know your priorities when it comes to (1) niche, (2) ideal student, and (3) location.

In my example about moving my classes to another city, I had decided that "ideal student" was the most important of the three to me.

So I defined my ideal student first, then I adjusted my teaching niches and my physical teaching location to match those students.

Of course, I could have instead chose location as the most important. I could have said, "I want to teach in Hillsboro where it's convenient to me." In that case, I would have adjusted my niche and ideal student to match those who lived in Hillsboro.

Or I could have taken "niche" (that is, the problems I solve or curiosities I satisfy for my students) and given it more prominence, then adjusted location and students to match.

For me though, I was – and still am - much more interested in the type of student I teach. I like working with certain types of students. So it makes sense for me to go where those ideal students are (location) and teach them what they want (niche). I always adjust my location and niche to match my priority, which is working with my ideal students.

Looking back, this choice of prioritizing "ideal student" led me in a directions I wouldn't have expected at the time.

As you saw earlier, it led me first to teaching in a city I hadn't previous considered. From there, my search for ideal students led me from being just a local teacher to an international teacher offering distance learning.

When I did that, "location" became even less of a concern.

Today, I'm in more niches now than ever, and teaching remotely through online courses, newsletters, and books.

But I still focus first and foremost on my "ideal students" and offering them what both they and I want to explore.

This book you are reading now is an example.

I have some "ideal students" who make up my private *Qi Masters* group. A good number of the members of that group are masters and instructors (or want to be instructors). They asked me to create some training on student attraction for them. Since I like to create training for my ideal students, I created first a video course, and then this book, for them.

With "ideal students" as my priority, I often do that. I find out what those ideal students want, and I give it to them.

But that's my choice. Your priority may be totally different. There are no right and wrong answers here when it comes to choosing priorities. You have to know yourself, and what would make you happy as a Tai Chi and Qigong teacher.

Implementing Your Priority

Of course, you can also always reconsider and change priorities. But making an initial commitment to one of these options will make the process easier.

You have to decide which is most important to you: *niche, ideal student,* or *location.*

If you decide niche is most important, look for students and locations that match.

For example, let's say your niche priority is that you like *helping martial artists add "soft skills" to their self-defense practices through Tai Chi and Qigong.*

In that case, your "ideal students" may be those who are already participating in karate, tae kwan do, muy thai, or some other "hard" martial arts.

So where would you look for locations?

Well, in your local area, you might check out martial arts schools where you could teach workshops or ongoing classes to their existing students.

If you want to go more national or international, you might check out martial arts associations, especially those that hold yearly conventions. You could do workshops at these conventions. Teaching workshops like that also helps you connect with other martial art schools that might be willing to sponsor workshops in other cities around the country, or around the world.

If you decide ideal student is most important, look for niches and locations to match.

This is exactly what I've done. So the experience I shared earlier about searching for a location is a good model to follow. Start with a strong description of a *student avatar,* and look for locations where you might find students like your avatar.

If you decide location is most important, look for niches and students to match.

You might decide this especially if you live in a small town and you really want to just be a local teacher helping people in your community. So you're going to need to look for niches and students to match what the community wants.

In the chapter on *Finding Your Teaching Niches,* I already gave you ideas on how to find a niche using my "two list" method. Well, when you create List #2 (the "what others want" list), just focus that list on your local community.

Other ways you can get ideas about niches and ideal students is to research the demographics of the city or region you are in. Find out the population size, the ages, the number of children, the income, and other information like that which can give you clues to what your local community might want.

That research is easy to do these days online. A few web searches using the name of your city plus adding a key word like *population, median income, age,* or even *demographics* can give you most of the answers you need.

Another way to do this demographic research is to spend time in the area. Driving around the area, looking at the homes and businesses, can often produce some good observations.

For example, once I identified Lake Oswego as a place to find my ideal students, I drove around the city. That's how I found that health food store with the fitness center.

Spending time in the area is invaluable. Another one of my favorite research methods is to go to a local coffee shop, preferably one that's busy, and just sit and listen to the conversations around me. I've actually gotten ideas for courses that I've taught to my students based on topics I over-heard in coffee shops.

Also, talk to people in the community. You don't have to talk to them about Tai Chi or Qigong. Just find out what their problems are, what their concerns are, and what they are interested in. Even if their answers are completely off the topic of Tai Chi and Qigong, they may have problems you could help solve with Tai Chi and Qigong. Those would also make good ideas for niches to match the location.

Know Your Priorities

The important point here though is to know your priorities.

Decide for yourself which is most important to you – *niche, ideal student,* or *location* – and then adjust the other factors to match.

Virtual Locations

For most of this chapter, we've focused mostly on how to research geographic locations. That fits best with what most instructors are interested in – teaching in-person classes or workshops in their local community, or maybe national or international workshops.

But if you teach primarily through distance learning using online courses, books, videos, newsletters, etc., then *virtual location* can be just as important.

Instead of finding people in the "real world," you are finding people where they are in the "virtual world."

For online teachers, your location focuses on *where you are likely to find new students through online media.*

It becomes about finding students on social media, on forums, through online searches, on blogs, and on media sites like video sharing sites.

Now, with many of these sites and with other online tools, you can get access to demographics for website visitors. Just like the geographic demographics I showed you earlier for those Oregon cities, these online demographics can be just as important and just as helpful.

Also, if you have your own website, you can often get similar demographics for your website visitors, especially those signing up for your email list or buying your courses and programs. You can get demographic information for them too, usually through your web host or other online tools.

You want to place online ads where you are more likely to find your ideal students. Because even if you teach remotely through books, video, or online, you may find that geographic location plays a greater role than you might expect. There may be parts of your country, or parts of the world, that respond more to what you offer than others, even if you are an online instructor.

For example, I've never had a student sign up for one of my online courses from North Dakota here in the U.S. It could be because of the relatively small population, or because of the interests of the people there, but I've never taught a North Dakotan. As a result, I long ago stopped advertising my online courses to those in North Dakota. It doesn't appear that my students are there.

On the other hand, I wind up getting a lot of registrations from places like California, Illinois (especially around Chicago), Florida, and Texas. So those are places where demographics are important to me.

I also get quite a few members from Canada, Australia, and the United Kingdom. Plus I get members from almost every European country, so demographics are important there for me too. The only notable exception in Europe is Germany. For some reason, few of my ideal students are there. But they are in France, Spain, Norway, Sweden, and Switzerland.

As you work through your location research, you'll find geographic locations that are more important or less important to you, even if you are not a geographically-bound teacher.

Moving Forward

I suggest that you spend some time thinking about your own priorities when it comes to *niche, ideal student,* and *location.* Decide which one is <u>your</u> priority.

Also, I'd suggest getting some practice doing location research.

In previous chapters, you identified your niches and created some ideal students. With those two pieces of the "Student Attraction" puzzle in mind, take some time to brainstorm to find locations where you might find those niches and ideal students.

I understand that if you decide location is your priority, you may want to change your niche and ideal student to match. But for now, don't worry about that. Just get some experience with *location research* using the niches and avatars you already have.

So take your niches and avatars, and identify some possible locations you think might work.

Once you have those locations, do some research on the demographics of those locations. Use the city demographics we discussed earlier in this chapter as a model - age, population growth, income, households, and children. Add in any other criteria that are relevant to your niche and ideal students, such as education level, gender, nationality, hobbies, interests, etc.

Once again, online resources are an easy way to do this research.

As I mentioned earlier, you could go to a search engine and enter *demographics* plus the city name – for example: *demographics Portland Oregon*.

Or you could put in *Portland Oregon income* to get income figures. So use your online resources to do some demographic research.

If you can, after you've done some brainstorming and done some demographic research, visit the location. Drive and walk around. Observe the people. Go into the shops. Eat in the restaurants. Spend time at the local coffee shop.

Do all of this to try to get a sense of the people that live and work there, and to see if the location matches where your ideal students might be.

Here's what's important: Don't worry about getting this location research perfect. Just get practice doing it. The more you do this sort of demographic research, the easier it becomes.

Action Items

Note: Make sure you complete these action items before moving on to the next chapter.

Find Where My Ideal Students Are

For each niche and avatar from the previous steps:

- Brainstorm locations (cities, facilities) where I might find my ideal students
- Research online to see if the demographics of these locations might match my avatars.

- Make a list of locations that match.
- If possible, after brainstorming and research, visit the locations:
  - Drive and walk around.
  - Observe the people, visit the shops, eat at restaurants, and visit coffee shops
  - Do these people seem to match the general characteristics of my avatar?
- Don't worry about getting this research perfect – just get it done!

Offering Your Students What They Want

Back in the 1990's, U.S. public television had featured a prime-time special on Qigong. For a few months after that, you couldn't open a magazine or newspaper without finding an article or news story about Qigong.

At the time, I was a brand new Qi instructor, teaching for those hospital fitness centers that I mentioned in the last chapter. All of a sudden, thanks to that TV show and all the media hype, we had hundreds of people signing up for Tai Chi and Qigong classes.

Two years earlier, the health center where I taught offered only two beginning classes, taught by one teacher. But not too long after this media hype, we were offering twelve beginning classes and six advanced classes, employing three teachers, including me.

Each beginning class had thirty or forty people in it. So we had around 400 or so beginners that term, with several dozen more on our wait list.

But none of these students really knew what Tai Chi or Qigong were about.

The media sensationalized Qigong, and these people were chasing that sensation.

Most showed up at the first class expecting they'd learn to throw people across the room without touching them, as was demonstrated on the TV show. Or they expected to learn to heal cancer, diabetes, and any other disease, all just using their mind. At least one new student told me he wanted to learn how to float in the air.

Of course, what happened as soon as they found out what it really takes to develop qi?

Yes, you guessed it. Most never came to a second class, once they had to actually do exercises.

"I didn't know I'd have to do any exercising. I thought this was all done with your mind," said one student at the end of his first – and only - class.

The other problem with all of the media hype?

Several students – who had never been to a Qigong or Tai Chi class ever before in their lives – told me that I wasn't teaching it properly. They told me that they had watched that TV show, and what I was doing wasn't on the show. So they said that apparently I didn't really know Qigong.

Student Expectation Problems

Now I often tell this story as an example of what happens during those brief periods of time when Tai Chi or Qigong becomes "popular" or becomes a "fad."

If you are not careful, you wind up with a lot of people in your classes who don't seriously want to learn. They just want to be part of the fad.

But this story also points out the problems teachers have with new student expectations.

Even when Tai Chi and Qigong aren't fads, rarely does a new student walk into your class <u>purely</u> to learn Tai Chi and Qigong, for the sake of those arts.

Instead, the vast majority are there because they want to get something from learning Tai Chi and Qigong.

For example, they may have had a few falls, and they are looking for better balance. They may have arthritis, and they are looking for better mobility. They may be martial artists, and they are looking to add some qi skills to their self-defense practice. They may be stressed, and they are looking for a way to unwind.

These are just a few of hundreds of examples of the reasons a new student might be in your class. And there's where expectation problems begin, if you are not careful in how you describe what you teach.

Let's say you advertised that you teach Tai Chi or Qigong, with an ad like this one:

"Beginners Tai Chi, Mondays at 6:30pm. Come join us to learn this ancient art for health, relaxation, and self-defense."

Or maybe it just says,

"Beginners Tai Chi, Mondays at 6:30pm."

Well, here's what happens in the minds of prospective students when they see and read an ad like that.

They think, *"Hey, I heard that Tai Chi is good for X,"* where X is a problem they have or a curiosity they'd like to explore.

So they fill in the blank you left in your offer. They think, *"Tai Chi is good for X, and here's a Tai Chi class, so if I go to this class, I'll get X."*

The Start of Retention Problems

Of course, you may or may <u>not</u> offer their particular X. So what happens when you don't make explicit what you <u>do</u> offer? You get a dozen new students, who all have different X's. Every single person there will have different expectations of what they'll get out of your class.

Of course, it's not possible for one teacher to meet such widely differing expectations. You couldn't even if you wanted. No teacher can be all things to all students.

But this is not just about expectations. This is also where retention problems start.

Students who don't get their expectations met will eventually quit your class.

Seems obvious, doesn't it?

They wanted X, you don't teach X, so they leave. If you are lucky, they'll just drop out of your class. If you are unlucky, they'll want refunds, they'll tell their friends how bad your class was, or they'll post bad reviews online.

This happens <u>not</u> because you aren't a good teacher, but simply because they had expectations, and you failed to meet them.

The Solution to a High Drop-out Rate

So what's the solution? You have to identify those expectations <u>before</u> the prospect signs up for your class. You should make sure they know whether your class meets their expectations or not <u>before</u> they register.

So how do you do that?

One solution is to pre-screen students.

For example, most teachers allow anyone to register. They don't pre-screen students to see if their class and their teaching approach are right for the student. They also don't find out if the student is right for the teacher – that is, if he or she is the kind of student they work best with.

Instead, they allow anyone to register ... and that's a sure fire recipe for a high drop-out rate.

You are allowing students who have a high probability of dropping out to register. So it should be no surprise when they do eventually drop out.

Now, some teachers try to solve this problem "after the fact." They allow anyone to register, but then they try to set the expectations of the students in the first class. In the first session, they'll cover what Tai Chi and Qigong are about, what the class is about, and what the students can expect to get out of the class.

But by that point, it's too late. You aren't <u>setting</u> their expectations at that point. Instead, you've already begun <u>disappointing</u> them.

You are already failing to meet the expectations the prospect has been carrying with them since before they signed up.

Instead of setting expectations, you are just giving them reasons to quit.

The solution? Before they register, let them know what your class is all about.

Setting Expectations Before They Register

Of course, you can do that with a screening process. You could meet with new students or talk to them on the phone before they register. You can ask them about their interests, and see if you have a match before taking their registration.

You can do this informally, or you could even have a more formal application process, where they complete an application and have an interview with you before accepting their registration.

I did both of these early on, and they were helpful. But later, I found that there's an <u>easier</u> way to do screening that requires less work and intervention on your part.

You can have the prospective student <u>screen themselves</u>.

It's actually easy to do, much easier than you might guess.

All that you need to do is make it clear what the students can expect from your class right from the start. Then when your prospective students find out about your class, they will screen themselves "out" if their expectations don't match, or screen themselves "in" and register if they do.

You can set these student expectations from the <u>first point of contact</u> they make with you.

It doesn't matter how you get new students.

If you get new students by advertising, you can set expectations in the first ad they see. If they find you online through your website or through social media, you'll set expectations on your website or your social media page.

If you do offline ads, like flyers posted in your community or course descriptions in community brochures, you can set those expectations in your flyers and descriptions.

No matter how students find you, you can set those expectations and have students self-screen themselves, right from that first point of contact.

Here's an example of setting expectations for this self-screening.

Let's say instead of offering *"Beginners Tai Chi, Mondays at 6:30pm"* like most ads do, your ad says *"Improve Your Balance to Prevent Falls with Tai Chi, Mondays at 6:30pm."*

What happens is that the students who wanted Tai Chi to help them with their arthritis, with their self-defense, or with relaxation, will most likely <u>ignore</u> your offer.

They'll think something like, *"Hey, I heard Tai Chi is good for throwing people across the room, but this class is about improving balance. It's probably not for me."*

But the prospective students <u>with</u> balance problems?

They'll be the ones who sign up for your class and will stick with it.

You'll most likely wind up with a room full of students that are fairly close to your ideal student.

You've successfully let the students self-screen themselves, all from simply making sure that your "offer" clearly sets expectations.

Becoming a Problem Solver

To do this, we may need to make another mindset shift.

I know that we usually think of ourselves as Qi instructors. But to be successful at student attraction and retention, from this day forward, you need to stop thinking of yourself as a "Qigong instructor" or a "Tai Chi teacher."

Instead, you need to think of yourself as *an instructor who solves problems and satisfies curiosities, but who just happens to use Qi practices to do the 'solving' and 'satisfying.'*

Or to put this another way …

> **Look at yourself, think about yourself, and really get a feel for yourself as someone who <u>first and foremost</u> is offering to <u>solve problems</u> and <u>satisfy curiosities</u> that your prospective students have.**

Tai Chi and Qigong are the means you use to do that, but they are <u>NOT</u> what you offer your students.

You don't offer Tai Chi or Qigong. Instead, you offer to solve their problems or satisfy their curiosities.

The Power of the Right Offer

This is where all of the work you've done in finding your niche, identifying your ideal students, and finding the right location now pays off.

You can offer students what they want, because you know their problems and curiosities.

You identified those problems and curiosities by finding your teaching niche. You narrowed it down even more when you put together your ideal student avatar. And during your location research, you found out more about the types of people who have those problems or curiosities.

So there's no guesswork here at this point. You know what to offer them.

Your course title, your course description, your advertising, your website, your social media pages, your flyers, your brochures, even your "phone script" when you talk to students who call – you make sure all of it is written to your ideal student. You write and speak in a way that attracts that sort of student to you.

To do that, you focus on the types of problems you can solve and the curiosities you can satisfy for them.

**Because you are no longer offering them
"just" Tai Chi or "just" Qigong.**

You are offering them solutions.

Talk About the Crabgrass

There's an old bit of advice that is given to people who work in sales: *"When you talk to customers, don't tell them about your weed killer. Talk to them about their crabgrass."*

That is, don't talk to customers about your product or service. Instead, talk to them about their problems. Let them know you understand their difficulties, and that you might be able to help them.

So we can update that old advice for ourselves:

"Don't tell new students about your Qigong or Tai Chi. Tell them that you know about their problems - and that you have a way to help them."

In the next chapter, we'll go into detail into the most important way you can do this. It's the single most powerful way you can get your solution across to attract your ideal students. It's the right way to present your offer so they know why they should sign up for your class, and keep coming back for more.

That will be in the next chapter. But for now, I'd like you to spend some time thinking about <u>what to offer</u> to your niches and your ideal students

The Right Title

Specifically, just for some practice with this mindset, I'd like to try a little experiment.

Using the niches and ideal student profiles you created in our previous chapters, I'd like you to come up with a <u>title</u> for the classes you would teach to each niche and ideal student in the niche.

To help you with this, here are a few examples.

Example 1: Tai Chi for Balance

Here's an example I gave earlier.

Let's say my niche is about helping people improve their balance, especially if they've already fallen or have a fear of falling.

If that's the case, I would definitely <u>NOT</u> call my class *"Beginners Tai Chi."*

Instead, I might call it ...

"Improve Your Balance to Prevent Falls with Tai Chi"

... or ...

"Prevent Falls with Tai Ch,"

... or maybe ...

"Better Balance with Tai Chi."

Those titles certainly do a better job of explaining what my class would be about.

It will also do a better job of attracting my ideal students, much better than if I just call my class *"Beginners Tai Chi."*

Example 2: Qigong for Arthritis

If my niche was using Wild Goose Qigong to help arthritis patients gain mobility, I <u>wouldn't</u> call my course *"Beginning Wild Goose Qigong."*

I wouldn't even call it *"Qigong for Arthritis."*

Instead I would call it:

"Regain Your Mobility Back From Arthritis with Qigong."

That title focuses on the problem my ideal students would like to solve.

Example 3: Tai Chi for Martial Arts

If I taught martial artists how to use Tai Chi for self-defense, I <u>wouldn't</u> call my course *"Beginning Tai Chi"* or even *"Tai Chi for Self-Defense."*

I would call it …

"Boost Your Martial Power with Tai Chi"

… or …

"Defend Yourself with the Power of Qi."

... or maybe even ...

"Becoming a 'Qi Warrior' with Tai Chi"

Once again, these course titles speak directly to my ideal students and their curiosity about martial Tai Chi.

Example 4: Qi For Cancer Recovery

If I taught cancer recovery patients how to get back some of their energy after chemo-therapy, I would call my course ...

"Revitalize Your New Cancer-Free Life with Qigong"

... or ...

"Energize Your Cancer Recovery with Tai Chi."

These titles are niche-focused and student-focused. They are better than a vague title like "Qigong for health."

Focus Your Course Title on the Offering

These are just examples that I've done off the top of my head. I could probably come up with better names if I actually explored the niche and came up with the right student avatars and location information.

But you get the idea.

Instead of focusing on what is being taught, each <u>title</u> focuses on the <u>problem</u> or <u>curiosity</u>.

You'll notice that most of these course titles follow a specific format. They are usually something like:

[Action verb] your [desired benefit or result] with [Tai Chi, Qigong, Qi, etc.]

Most of the examples above start with an action verb like *improve, prevent, boost, regain, defend, revitalize, energize,* etc. Then a desired benefit or result follows: *balance, mobility, martial power, recovery,* etc. It's only when you get to the end of the title that we mention Tai Chi or Qigong.

Your Turn

Now that you have this format and have seen my examples, it's your turn.

I'd like you to do the same for all the niches and ideal student avatars you've already created. Come up with a course title for each one – a title that would attract that ideal student, because it shows you understand their problem and can help them with it.

Use the examples we've covered here as models for the titles of your own course offering.

In the next chapter, I'll show an even more effective way to present what you offer to new and existing students. But having these course titles is the first step.

So for now, start with these course titles to help get you into your new "student attraction and retention" mindset.

Action Items

Note: Make sure you complete these action items before moving on to the next chapter.

<u>Offer My Students What They Want</u>

For each niche and avatar from the previous steps:

- Create a "course title" to offer for each.
- For the title/offer, <u>don't</u> focus just on what is being taught (e.g., Tai Chi, Qigong, styles).
- Focus more on the problem or curiosity this niche and avatar have.
- Use the examples given in this chapter. Most titles follow this format: "[action verb] your [desired benefit or result] with [Tai Chi, Qigong, Qi, etc.]"
- Don't worry about being perfect with this — just get it done.

Developing Your Unique Learning Proposition

I'd like you to take a few moments, and imagine the following scenario.

But don't just read my description of this scene passively.

Really imagine it.

Using the full power of your imagination, please visualize, think about, and get a strong feeling for this scene, as if it were actually happening to you right now.

What Would You Say?

Let's imagine that you're in your teaching location, and you're about to begin a new session of classes.

A prospective Qi student, someone you don't know and who doesn't know you, has walked into your classroom. He has arrived before you've started the class and before anyone else has arrived. He is considering whether or not to register for your class, and he wants know more about what you teach.

But there's a catch in this scenario.

When the new, prospective student walks up to you, you are allowed to say <u>only one sentence</u> to him.

That's all – just one sentence.

131

After hearing that one sentence, the prospective student will decide either to (a) stay and register for the class, based on that sentence, or (b) decide not to register for your class, and leave to go look for another Qi class.

What one sentence would you say to him?

Helping With Their Decision

Now, to make this clear ...

For this scenario, you are <u>not</u> trying to manipulate him into joining. You are <u>not</u> trying to tell him what he wants to hear to get him to join. You are <u>not</u> trying to trick him into registering.

Instead, you are trying to make sure the new student gets as <u>much</u> info about your class as you can <u>cram</u> into one sentence.

This sentence should help him make a good decision about whether your class is right <u>or not</u> for what he is looking for. Your goal with this sentence is to make sure he registers <u>if and only if</u> the class is right for him.

You may have heard the saying, *"You never get a second chance to make a first impression."* This sentence will be your first impression.

You want to make it a strong one that really puts forth exactly why this student should register with you, but only <u>if</u> you really are the right teacher for him.

I'd like you to take a moment, right now, to come up with the one sentence you would say to this potentially new student. Craft a sentence that would help him make the right decision both for himself as a student and for you as his possible teacher.

Stop reading, put this book down, and create your sentence right now.

Where We Started

When we started this book on student attraction and retention, we identified the two biggest problems in those areas today.

They were:

- *Competition* – Today's prospective students have more options for learning than they ever have had in the history of Tai Chi and Qigong. How can you compete with all of these options to attract students?

- *Conflicting Student Expectations* - Every student walks into your class expecting to get something out of it, but students can have widely varying expectations. It's not possible for one teacher to meet such widely differing expectations, which leads to problems with student retention.

To help with these problems, we've been exploring a Zero Drop Outs Strategy to deal with these problems. So far, we've gotten through four of the five steps:

- ✓ Find your teaching niches.

- ✓ Identify your ideal students.

- ✓ Find out where those students are.

- ✓ Find out what those students want.

These four steps fix many attraction and retention problems. But our fifth step is the "secret sauce" that takes everything we've done to a higher level.

That fifth step is:

- ✓ Make sure those students know <u>why</u> they should be <u>your</u> students.

Sealing the Deal

While the first four steps can go a long way to improving your attraction and retention, this fifth step often seals the deal.

That's because an iron-clad way to pull in new students - once you've identified who they are and what they want - is to offer them a <u>special reason</u> to become <u>your</u> student.

You need to give them something that:

- ✓ Speaks directly to their problems or curiosities,

plus …

- ✓ Gives them a unique reason why they should sign up with you, and not someone else.

So how do you do this? How do you let students know why they should be <u>your</u> students, and no one else's?

Just answer this question:

> *"Of all the options that your prospective students have available to them, why should they choose <u>you</u> and <u>your</u> class?"*

As we said, your prospects have all kinds of options for learning Tai Chi and Qigong. So what is <u>different</u> about your class? And not just different, but what is <u>compelling</u> about your class?

Or to put this question another way:

> *"What's so special about learning Tai Chi or Qigong from <u>you</u> rather than anyone else?"*

If you do <u>not</u> have answers to these questions, attraction and retention will be an ongoing problem.

But if you <u>can</u> answer these questions, you may never have to worry about competition or conflicting student expectations ever again.

It's Your ULP

Ideally, you should be able to answer these questions with <u>just one sentence</u>.

Your one sentence should answer these questions with a unique and compelling reason that speaks directly to the type of students you want.

It has to be a compelling reason <u>not</u> just to learn Tai Chi or Qigong, but to learn it from <u>you</u>. It has to be something that they might be able to get <u>only</u> from you.

It can't be something they believe they can get from another teacher in town, from free online videos, or from yoga or other exercises.

You have to give them a unique reason to come to <u>your</u> class and study with <u>you</u> versus every other option they have available to them.

We call this reason a *"ULP."*

That stands for *"unique learning proposition."*

It's a statement about what they can learn only from you and from no one else. It's a statement that distinguishes you from other teachers. It's the reason for them to choose you over all of their other options for learning Tai Chi and Qigong.

You are offering to them a unique learning opportunity, and your *"ULP sentence"* describes that opportunity.

Weak ULPs

You may be wondering, *"How can I be unique as a teacher, or offer a unique class? I teach the same styles and forms that other teachers teach."*

Well, let's start with what is <u>not</u> a good *"Unique Learning Proposition."*

First of all, a ULP should <u>never</u> be about the style you teach. Most styles aren't unique. They aren't something only you teach.

This is why, even though my beginning class is *Eight Brocades Qigong,* you never see me call the class *"Eight Brocades Qigong."* Teaching *Eight Brocades* is not unique. A lot of teachers teach it. So *Eight Brocades* would not make a good ULP.

Of course, maybe you do teach a rare or unique style, one that no one else teaches. Even if that's the case, a ULP about your style is usually a weak ULP. While your style may be unique, it's usually <u>not</u> compelling enough, especially to beginning students. Over time, they may learn to care about how your style is unique, but that usually doesn't happen up front. That's usually not going to attract prospective students to your class at the start.

That's a mistake many Tai Chi and Qigong teachers make. They try to attract students with something like style. That really isn't compelling enough to a prospective student.

Lineage is another example.

You see teachers struggle when they try to use their lineage as a way to attract students.

A lineage isn't compelling enough for a ULP. This might be hard to swallow, especially if you're a lineage teacher. But most new students don't care who your teacher was, or if you can trace your lineage back a thousand years.

Look at it and think about it this way. The vast majority of students don't one day out of the blue wake up and say ...

"Well, what I really want from Tai Chi is to know that my teacher's teacher's teacher's teacher was some old guy known only to five people in 1800's China."

I'm not saying there isn't anyone like that. But usually, that type of specialized curiosity comes only from students who have <u>already</u> been studying Tai Chi or Qigong for a while. That often will be a very small niche of students, and they may be difficult to find. So a lineage-based ULP won't attract many students.

You also see teachers try to attract new students based on "specialized styles," like *senior's tai chi* or *tai chi for arthritis*.

As we mentioned in the chapter on niches, these categories are far too broad. So they aren't compelling enough on their own to be a ULP. After all, just because your prospects are the same age, or have the same disease, doesn't mean they will all have the same expectations when they walk into your class. So you are setting yourself up for retention problems if that's what you are using to attract students.

Other weak attraction methods you sometimes see teachers use are based on things like "teaching quality."

They try to attract students by talking about how good of a teacher they are, or about how much more effective their approach is. Or they try to use their credentials or what certificates they've earned. These examples are all weak student attraction approaches, too.

Now, I'm not saying you shouldn't have credentials, or teach as part of a lineage, or teach seniors, or teach those who have arthritis, or be more effective.

All of those things are great characteristics to have in place to <u>support</u> your Unique Learning Proposition. You might even include some of them in your ULP sentence, but they are never the main feature.

Making a Better ULP

First and foremost, a good ULP has to be from the prospective student's point of view. It has to be something she can immediately tune into and see herself in.

Things like styles, credentials, lineage – students won't see themselves in that, not at first. It's not personal enough.

> **A good ULP has to be about the students' wants, <u>not</u> about what you think is important or what you think they need.**

A ULP has to immediately grab the prospect within just a few seconds, and make them say, *"Hey, I haven't seen something like this before, but it might just be for me."*

ULP Examples

To give you an idea of how this works for Qi teachers, let me give you a few examples of this right now.

And to make this as real as possible for you, I'm going to be using examples from *my own* courses, books, and programs. If you've been with me in my courses for any length of time, you may have seen some or all of these ULPs in action.

These are the *one sentence ULPs* I've used for my courses.

Example #1: Health, Stress Relief, Qi

You are About to Discover How to Improve Your Health, Relieve Stress, and Develop Chi in Just 10 Minutes a Day with the "Chi" Secrets to Tai Chi and Qigong.

Example #2: Chi Boost

Give Yourself a "Chi Boost" - Three-Time Hall-of-Fame Master Divulges His Easiest and Fastest "Chi Life Energy" Techniques to Give You a Quick Boost to Improve Your Health, Relieve Stress, and Feel Great.

Example #3: Tai Chi Theory

"De-Mystify" Your Tai Chi and Qigong - Three-Time Hall-of-Fame Master Pulls Back the Curtain to Reveal the "Secret Chi Theory" Behind Tai Chi and Qigong in Practical, Everyday Language for Experienced Students and Instructors

Example #4: Qi Masters

Discover the Secrets to Becoming a "Qi Master" ... How to Break Through to Higher Levels of Health, Stress Relief, Vitality, Energy, and Power in your Tai Chi and Qigong Practice

Example #5: Qi Student Attraction

Attention: Tai Chi and Qigong Instructors ... Fill Your Classes, Workshops and Programs with Dedicated, Enthusiastic Students, Cut Your Drop-Out Rate to Zero, and Attract New Students Like a Magnet - with this Five-Step Secret Strategy from a Hall-of-Fame Master

More Than Just A Headline

If you have been one of my students for any length of time, some or all of the five sentences I just gave you might sound familiar.

As a matter of fact, since you've purchased this book, you probably saw example #5 when you made your purchase. It's right on the back cover of this book, plus in the description part of the listings for the book online.

So you might recognize these examples as *headlines* that I've used on my websites and in some of my promotions for the courses, books, and programs I offer.

But these sentences are more than just headlines.

They are my ULPs.

If I could say only one sentence to a prospective student in each of my various niches, these would be the sentences I would say.

These sentences speak directly to my ideal student avatars in each niche, reinforcing the benefits they will receive from the course or program.

But What Is Unique?

Now, it's true that some of the benefits in my ULPs are <u>not</u> available from other teachers. That truly makes them <u>unique</u>.

But you may have noticed that some of the benefits in my ULPs actually <u>are</u> available from other teachers. For example, some of my ULPs mention "improving health" or "relieving stress." Many teachers make those same claims.

So what makes my ULPs unique then?

Well, your ULP doesn't have to be "unique" in the sense that it has never existed in the history of the world before.

It doesn't even have to be "unique" in the sense that no other teacher teaches it or teaches that way.

It just has to be unique to your prospective students. It may be something that the students may not have heard about from other teachers in the niche. Or it may be something other teachers offer, but you've expressed in a unique fashion – in a way that other teachers don't talk about it.

It has to be something that prospective students may have never seen before in the niche they are in, or at least expressed in a way they haven't heard before.

Other teachers might provide the same benefit, but if the other teachers <u>don't talk</u> about the benefit, or don't talk about it in the way you do, it will be unique to your prospects.

"But Everyone Does This!"

Let me give you an historical example of this. This is an example from <u>outside</u> of Tai Chi and Qigong.

This is a classic true story told in many marketing and business niches.

Back in the early 1900's in the U.S., Schlitz Brewery in Milwaukee, Wisconsin was struggling. They had fallen to fifth in overall sales behind some much bigger competitors in the beer market.

At the time, nearly all brewers were advertising their beer as "pure." Some were a bit vague about what that meant. But most advertising talked about the type of water the beer makers used in brewing, about their ingredients, about the filtering processes they used, or about the brewing process itself.

Just about every beer maker advertised themselves that way, because that's what the buying public wanted to know about their beer at that time. They wanted to know it was "pure."

Every brewery had different processes for making their beer pure. But they all talked about "purity" in their advertising, and they all talked about it in the same way. The advertising was all about their special ingredients or their filtration process.

Schlitz had also been advertising their purity, but their sales continued to fall. They were just another "me too" brewery in a crowded field of "pure" brewers.

So Schlitz hired a gentleman by the name of Claude Hopkins, a marketing specialist, to help them increase their sales through advertising.

When Hopkins toured the Schlitz Brewery, the brewers were showing him these same things that were in their ads – the different types of water, the ingredients, and the filtration process they used.

But during the tour, they passed by a room where Schlitz "steam-cleaned" their beer bottles. The tour guides were going right past the room, but Hopkins stopped and asked what was going on in there.

One of the brewers said, *"That's where we steam-clean our bottles, to make sure there is nothing to contaminate the beer when we put it into the bottles."*

Hopkins said, *"Well, I drink beer, but I've never heard of this. Why don't you talk about this in your ads?"*

The brewer said, *"But there's nothing special about that. Every brewer does it, and we all do it the same way."*

Hopkins said, *"Yes, but none of you are talking about it."*

So Hopkins created a new ad campaign. To emphasize Schlitz's commitment to purity, he created the tagline "Schlitz beer bottles - Washed with live steam."

That campaign helped propel Schlitz from fifth place in sales to first place in sales in just a few months.

The Lesson for Us

The lesson here for us, as Tai Chi and Qigong instructors, is that our "unique learning proposition" - our ULP - doesn't have to be something only we do. That would be ideal, but it's not necessary.

It just has to be something that no other instructor in your niche and location is talking about.

Of course, we have an even bigger advantage here than Schlitz did, because we are Qi instructors and not brewers. The advantage is that _few_ Tai Chi and Qigong teachers create ULPs - or even figure out niches, student avatars, or locations, for that matter.

As a result, it's relatively easy for us to stand out from the crowd right now and develop a ULP. We can find a lot of things in our teaching to talk about that aren't necessarily "unique," but that _few_ instructors are talking about.

While they are busy talking about their styles, their lineage, or their certifications, we can focus in our ULP on the problems we solve and curiosities we satisfy.

Doing that, we'll automatically be talking about the stuff prospective students _aren't_ hearing from other instructors.

That means that a teacher with almost any type of ULP will stand out – since none of the other instructors even have one.

As a result, you don't have to be great at creating a ULP for yourself.

For example, you might create a ULP that a "professional marketer" might consider weak. It might be a ULP that would not work in more competitive niches outside of Qigong or Tai Chi.

But because you are in the Qi arts, where <u>few</u> teachers have anything like a ULP, your ULP will give you a distinct advantage.

You don't have to have a "strong" ULP. Almost any ULP right now will work, since other instructors don't have them.

I can't stress enough this advantage that we have <u>right now</u> in this regard.

So you don't have to worry if you've never created a ULP before. You don't have to worry if you feel like you don't know what you are doing when creating your ULP. You also don't have to worry if you think you won't be good at this "ULP stuff."

You just have to try.

Just trying puts you ahead of just about every other Qi instructor today.

So how do you try? How do you go about crafting your unique learning proposition?

Crafting Your ULP

There are a lot of different methods for crafting ULPs.

As a matter of fact, in niches outside of Tai Chi and Qigong, instead of "ULP," this statement is called a USP – a unique *selling* proposition. So if you go online right now and search for "unique selling proposition," you may find dozens of methods for creating a USP.

You can take any of those methods, replace the word "selling" with the word "learning," and the method will usually work in order to create a Tai Chi or Qigong ULP.

But I have a particular method I like to use when I need to create a ULP. I think it's one of the easiest methods. It's the one I tend to use the most.

Let me walk you through that method right now. It has only two steps.

ULP Step 1: Brainstorm

Step one of this method is to do some brainstorming.

Specifically, you'll want to brainstorm the features and benefits your "offer" provides to your niche, ideal student, and location.

By *offer*, I'm referring to the course and course titles you came up with in the last chapter. Those courses are your offers.

So for each course you offer, you want to identify the <u>features</u> and <u>benefits</u> of that offer.

By the way, you may not be familiar with the terms *feature* and *benefit*.

- A *feature* is an aspect of what you offer in your course.

- A *benefit* refers to how a particular feature <u>helps</u> your ideal student.

I'll walk through examples of both features and benefits in a moment.

But to make sure you have the process down, you'll want to make a list of all the features plus their benefits.

These can be *direct benefits* of participating in the class – something that the class actually offers.

But you can also include *indirect benefits,* such as if there is a benefit to the location where you'll teach. Or if there are benefits to the method you'll use to deliver to the class. It could also be a benefit to the class structure and organization. It can also be benefits based on you, your relevant experience (if you are a member of the niche), your background, or your certification.

You'll want to list as many *features* and *benefits* as you possibly can. I try to list at least fifteen to start with.

If you are having trouble coming up with this list, but you already teach, you have an advantage. You have a group of people you can ask. You can ask your students why they were attracted to your class, and why they keep coming back. Often times, you'll find features and benefits you may not have even thought of by asking your students why they are there.

But let's say you don't have students to ask, and you need to brainstorm this yourself.

Let me go through an example to help you. I'm going to start with an offer or course title I mentioned in the last chapter.

Offer: Improve Your Balance with Tai Chi

Features/Characteristics	Benefits
Improves balance	Prevents falling, removes worry about hurting yourself from falls.
Better mobility	Can get around more easily, perform daily tasks, easier to stand and walk.
Short 9-movement form	Easy to learn, can be learned in a few weeks, not much memorization.
Can be practiced in a small area	Don't need special location to practice, can be done anywhere even in a small

	bedroom, especially in senior living spaces.
Can be done in 8 minutes	Fits into busy schedule, doesn't require a large commitment.
5 week course – 1 hour per week	Doesn't take much time to learn, can see benefits more quickly.
My certification	Only certified instructor in area, increases trust in getting results.
Have already taught this to 200 people	Have helped many students, so I know I can help you.
I have balance problems	I know this works, because it helped me, and since I have the same problems, I can help you better than someone who doesn't.

Let's say my offer – my course title – is *Improve Your Balance with Tai Chi.*

One of the features or characteristics for this course is obvious. The course improves balance. So I wrote that under the *Features* column of the list above.

So if *improves balance* is the feature, what benefits does that provide? Well, improved balance may prevent falls, plus it also removes the worries students may have about hurting themselves from falls. So those are two benefits that the feature of *improving balance* provides. I wrote those in the *Benefits* column in the above list.

The course might also help people with *better mobility.* That's the feature. So what benefits does better mobility provide?

I thought of three benefits to this off the top of my head. First, my students could get around more easily. Second, they can perform daily tasks more easily. Finally, they can also stand and walk around with greater ease when they have better mobility. Those are three benefits to the feature of better mobility.

Let's say that in this course, I'll be teaching a *short, nine-movement Tai Chi form.* Again, that's a feature of the course. So what are the benefits?

Well, because the form is short, it's easy to learn. It can be learned in just a few weeks. Plus it doesn't require much memorization. That's especially helpful if your ideal student is a senior, who doesn't have the patience or the memory capacity to remember a lot of complicated movements. Those are all benefits to learning a short form.

Let's say the form *can be practiced in a small area.* That feature means that you don't need a special location to practice. The form can be done anywhere, even in a small bedroom. That's especially helpful if your ideal student is a senior, who may reside in senior living. Sometimes, space is at a premium in their rooms, their apartments, or their condos. So that's another benefit to being able to practice in a small area.

Let's say another feature is that the form *can be done in about eight minutes.* Well, since it also doesn't require a large commitment in practice time, it would be easier to fit into a busy schedule.

Another feature may be that you teach a *five week course, one hour a week.* The benefit is that this form doesn't take much time to learn, and you can start to see improvements in balance more quickly than in longer forms of Tai Chi.

Let's say another feature is that you are *certified in teaching* this Tai Chi style, and indeed you are the only person certified in your area. That feature alone can help increase your students' trust in you and in the fact that they will get results from the course.

You may also have *already taught this course* to two hundred other students. With that, you can honestly say that you have helped many students, so you know you can help your ideal student too.

Finally, let's also say that *you yourself have had balance problems,* and you have been helped by this Tai Chi form. The benefits here are obvious. You know the form works, because it helped you. You can also better help others with balance problems, because you know what they are going through. You've been there yourself.

Now as I said, I usually like to list fifteen of these features or characteristics of the course, and then list the benefits associated with each feature.

But for this example, let's go ahead and stick with the nine features I've just listed here, along with their benefits.

ULP Step 2: Create Your ULP Statement

Once you have your list of features and benefits, step two of this process is to look for unique benefits – or a unique combination of benefits – that fits certain criteria.

Now remember, we are talking about *unique within the niche, ideal student, and location.*

It might not be unique in the sense of "never seen before," but at least unique in the sense of "never seen before by these ideal students in this niche at this location." You may not be the only one who provides these benefits, but you are the only one talking about it to your ideal students.

Here are the four criteria I use when I look for benefits for a ULP.

First, the benefit should be *important to your ideal student.*

If the benefit isn't important to your ideal students, that doesn't mean you won't provide the benefit when you teach. It just means you won't talk about it in your ULP. It will be more of a side benefit that they get from attending, not something you focus on in the ULP.

The second characteristic to look for is that the benefit can be *easily understood by your ideal student.*

Your course may have a benefit that takes some explaining to get the idea of the benefit across to your students. You may need three, four, or five sentences – or more – to explain the benefit. Something like that would not make a good benefit for your ULP. Everything in your ULP needs to be easily understood by your ideal student.

Now, some benefits might be easily understood by your ideal students, but not necessarily by <u>all</u> students or by anyone outside of your niche. If that's the case, it would <u>still</u> be a good benefit. As long as your ideal students understand it without a lot of explaining, you would use it in your ULP.

Another characteristic to look for is a benefit that is *difficult to find elsewhere by your ideal student.*

The key word is *"find."* It doesn't mean that other teachers don't offer the benefit. It just means they don't talk about it or promote it. So your ideal student might have a hard time finding it.

Ideally, one final characteristic for a good ULP benefit is that it is *difficult for other teachers to provide.*

That's not an absolute requirement here. You can have a benefit in your ULP that other teachers also provide. But if you do have a benefit that it would be hard for other teachers to provide, it should definitely be mentioned in your ULP.

So when you have your list of features and benefits, go through them looking for benefits that fit one or more of these criteria:

- Important to your ideal student.

- Easily understood by your ideal student.

- Difficult to find elsewhere by your ideal student.

- Difficult for other teachers to provide.

You'll want to find three to five benefits, or maybe more, that fit at least one or more of the above.

Once you have about three to five benefits like that, you just need to work those benefits into an action-oriented sentence to create your ULP.

Let's stick with the above example of an *"Improve Your Balance with Tai Chi"* course, and the nine features I listed above. Using that list, I've come up with five ULPs that would fit this course offering.

Take a moment to read through these ULPs. You'll see how I pulled various features and benefits to create each ULP.

I didn't always use the same features or benefits in each of these ULPs. I mixed them up a bit. In that way, you'll see how I worked a number of different benefits into these action-oriented ULPs.

Example #1:

Never Worry About Falling Again – Certified "Balance" Instructor Shows You How to Move Through Your Day with Greater Ease and Confidence in Just Eight Minutes a Day with Her Special "Tai Chi Balance" Approach

Example #2:

Better Balance in Eight Minutes a Day – Certified Tai Chi Instructor Shows You How to Prevent Falls, Walk More Easily, and Stand More Firmly With a Short Practice You Can Do Anytime, Anywhere.

Example #3:

Walk, Stand, and Sit With Ease – Certified Tai Chi Instructor (Who Overcame Her Own Balance Problems) Has Helped 200 Seniors With Her 8-Minute "Stability" Program, and She's Ready to Help YOU Overcome Your Fear of Falling.

Example #4:

Never Fall Again – A Short 8-Minute Tai Chi Routine from a Certified "Balance" Instructor (and a "Fall Survivor" Herself) Improves Balance, Speeds Recovery from Recent Falls, and Prevents Future Falls

Example #5:

You Are About to Discover The Easiest and Fastest Way to Remove the Fear of Falling Permanently, With a Simple 8-Minutes-a-Day "Tai Chi Balance" Routine That Can Be Practiced Anywhere, Anytime.

Using Your ULP

These would all be good ULPs for an *"Improve Your Balance with Tai Chi"* course.

Each of these would be a great "first sentence" to be used as headlines on your website, on your flyers, and in your brochures.

Any one of them could also be used as the first line of the description of your course if you advertise in a course catalog, say for your community parks and recreation department.

All of these ULPs would be great at attracting the ideal students in this niche to your course.

It's Your Turn

So now it's your turn.

As an exercise, take the niches, student avatars, and offers that you created in the previous chapters. Then do just what I did. List out your features and benefits for each course offering, and try to create one or more ULPs for that niche, student, and offer.

You can use all of the ULPs we covered in this chapter – both my own real ULPs, plus the ones I just did in the *"Tai Chi balance"* example – as models for your ULP.

Don't worry about making your ULPs perfect. Just get some practice going through this process.

You might struggle with the first few.

But after that, something will "click" within you, and crafting ULPs will become one of your strongest skills when it comes to attracting new students to your classes and programs.

Action Items

Note: Make sure you complete these action items before moving on to the next chapter.

<u>Develop my Unique Learning Proposition</u>

For each offer (course title) I've created:

- Write down a list with two columns:
    - Column #1 — Features/characteristics of the course
    - Column #2 — The benefits offered by the feature or characteristic in the first column.
- Come up with at least 15 features in column #1.
- From the column #2 <u>benefits</u>, choose 3 to 5 benefits with <u>one or more</u> of these criteria:
    - Important to my ideal student
    - Easily understood by my ideal student

- o Difficult to find elsewhere by my ideal student (not talked about by other teachers in the niche)
- o Difficult for other teachers to provide
- Turn these three to five benefits into a ULP:
  - o Work them into a single action-oriented statement.
  - o Think of this like a "first sentence" you could say to new students or a "headline" for your advertising.
  - o You may want to come up with several ULPs by mixing and matching different benefits.
  - o Use the examples provided in this chapter as models for your own ULPs.
- Don't worry about making the perfect ULP – just get some practice with it and get it done.

Recap: The Complete Zero Drop Outs Strategy

At this point, we've now completed our *Zero Drop Outs* "Student Attraction and Retention" Strategy.

To recap, the five steps of this strategy are:

1. Find your teaching niches.

2. Identify your ideal students.

3. Find out where those students are.

4. Find out what those students want.

5. Make sure they know why they should be your students.

Now that you know the details of each of these steps, we can summarize the Zero Drop Outs strategy with just five words:

1. Niche
2. Avatar
3. Location
4. Offer
5. ULP

Of course, there's more to having a successful class, program, or workshop than just these five steps.

So in our next chapter, we'll look at, talk about, and get a feel for the next steps you need to take. In these steps, you'll see how to create, promote, and deliver a new course or program that will ensure your success at attracting and keeping your ideal students.

Creating, Promoting, and Delivering Your Course

So far in this book, we've focused on a five step strategy for student attraction and retention. The five steps of this strategy were (1) niche, (2) avatar, (3) location, (4) offer, and (5) ULP.

We've spent a lot of time on these five steps for one primary reason. That is because of everything you could do while teaching Tai Chi and Qigong, these five steps will have the <u>biggest impact</u> on helping you to attract new students, and to retain them when you get them.

As you've seen and read about here, most problems with attraction and retention are solved <u>before</u> you or your students step foot in your classroom.

These five steps help you overcome the two biggest attraction and retention problems you face right at the start: *competition* and *conflicting student expectations*.

Lao Tzu, the ancient Chinese sage, said that *a journey of a thousand miles begins with a single step*. Well, the journey of teaching a Tai Chi or Qigong class begins with these five "student attraction" steps.

The *research and planning* in these steps makes sure you start your journey headed in the right direction.

The New Course Development Process

But as you might know, there's more to teaching a new course than just these research and planning steps. You have to create the course, promote it, and ultimately teach it to your new students.

I like to divide up the entire "new course development" process into six steps.

These steps are:

1. Research

2. Blueprint

3. Pricing Strategy

4. Promotion

5. Creation

6. Delivery

The first step in new course development is the *research* step. At this point, you <u>already know</u> how to research a new course. That was the focus of this book.

Our Zero Drop Outs Strategy describes the actual research I do when I create a new course, book, program, video, workshop, or membership group.

Once you have your niche, avatar, location, offer, and ULP, there's <u>no more</u> research you need to do at that point.

The remaining steps after the *research* step – *blueprint, pricing, promotion, creation, and delivery* - are a bit beyond the scope of this book. So we won't be diving into these steps in detail here.

But each of these additional steps <u>does</u> have certain aspects that are related to our primary discussion of finding and keeping new students.

So let's spend some time on the student attraction and retention topics related to each of these steps.

Blueprinting Your Offer

After the *research* step, the next step in the New Course Development Process is to *blueprint your offer.*

Blueprinting your offer means to create an overall plan for the program you'll be offering to teach.

To do that, you'll need to:

- Determine the details of the offer.

- Determine where and when the course will be held.

- Create a rough outline of the content of the course.

- Create a simple course description.

As we just said, there's a lot to consider in *blueprinting*, just like there is with all of the New Course Development steps. But for now, let's just focus on how *blueprinting* affects our main topics of student attraction and student retention.

Offer Details

First of all, you'll need to nail down the *details of the offer.*

Let's start with <u>how</u> you'll be delivering the program.

Is this delivered in-person, or is it done through remote teaching (online, video, book, etc.)? If it's in-person, is it a weekly class, a one-time workshop, a series of workshops, or one-on-one coaching?

If it's a class, will it be close-ended (that is, has a start date and end date, or meets for a finite number of sessions) or open-ended (starting on a certain date, but continuing on indefinitely)?

All of these choices have pro's and con's, and you need to make sure the choices fit your niche and ideal student.

For example, if you are going after new students who haven't studied with you previously, often times a close-ended offer that has a set number of sessions or set number of weeks attracts more students than an open-ended offer.

But if you are primarily targeting students who have studied with you before, often an open-ended offer will get you more registrations. Of course, this can vary from niche to niche, and from student avatar to student avatar.

In addition to delivery, group composition is another detail that needs to be identified.

Will this be a beginners-only class or a class of advanced students only? Will it be a mixed class of both beginners and advanced students?

Again, there are pro's and con's here as well.

For brand-new, never-studied-with-you-before students, a beginners-only class usually has better retention than a mixed class. However, depending on the niche and the offer, a mixed class may actually work out well for you.

Another detail you'll need is minimum and maximum numbers.

For the minimum, what is the least amount of students you'll need to have a viable class or program? At what number would the class become not worth your time to teach?

Also, what is the maximum number you can effectively teach? This number may be limited based on your own comfort with teaching large groups, but it may also be limited by the location and facility where you'll be teaching. But make sure you have a maximum number in mind as you blueprint your course.

Speaking of facility …

Schedule and Facility

As part of your blueprint, you'll also need to determine *when and where the course will be held.*

For in-person classes, these are important decisions.

Your schedule and your teaching facility must match the expectations of your ideal student avatar.

For example, if your ideal student is a senior citizen, night classes may <u>not</u> be a good choice when it comes to scheduling. Instead, a day class might be a better time for a senior's class, especially if your avatar is retired from work and has her days free.

On the other hand, if your avatar is a white-collar worker, classes during the 8 a.m. to 5 p.m. workday are often poor times. An after-work, evening schedule would be a better time.

Facility is important too. You need to hold your classes in a location that is likely to attract your ideal students.

For example, if you want to teach Tai Chi to young martial artists, a senior living facility may not be the best choice.

It <u>doesn't matter</u> if your location research shows that there are a lot of young martial artists in the area around the senior facility. Most of your target market won't even consider taking a Tai Chi class at a seniors' home, even if you try to explain to them the class really is for martial artists.

Of course, the opposite would also be true. If you want to teach seniors, most would be hesitant to sign up for a class at a karate dojo or kung fu school.

So you'll want to make sure your schedule and facility match your student avatar's expectations. Also, having the right facility may help expose your classes to potential students already at the facility.

For example, if you teach Tai Chi for martial artists at a martial arts school, you'll have a pool of martial artists already at that location who may be interested in your classes. The same is true if you teach seniors' Qigong at a senior living facility.

Course Outline

As part of your course blueprint, you'll also want a general outline of the content you'll be teaching.

You don't need to have every detail of what you'll be teaching planned out just yet, but you should have some bullet points or some key ideas about what the course will cover.

What's important here though is that outline of this content must show how you'll deliver on the *promise* made by your course title and your ULP. If you include a feature or benefit in your title or ULP, you have to be sure that the content of the course provides that feature or benefit.

If your course is entitled *Improve Balance with Tai Chi*, then your course content has to include exactly what you'll teach to improve balance.

If your ULP says that you are offering an *eight minute routine*, then your course has to teach an eight minute routine.

As you might imagine, <u>not</u> delivering on your course title or ULP will create retention problems.

Your outline can be short. Here's an example, using the same offering we used in our ULP chapter – that is, an *Improve Balance with Tai Chi* class.

<u>Improve Balance with Tai Chi – Outline</u>

This course will cover:

1. Posture
   a. Correct posture for Tai Chi and for daily life (within each person's limitations)
2. Upper body movement
   a. How to reach without overextending
   b. How to turn from neck, shoulders, and upper chest while maintaining balance
3. Lower body movement
   a. How to turn from the waist while keeping your balance
   b. How <u>not</u> to use the knees during turns (no knee twists)
   c. How to shift weight without shifting too much
4. Walking
   a. Posture during walking
   b. Toe direction as a guide
   c. Walk <u>without</u> falling into each step
5. "Tai Chi for Balance" short form
   a. All nine movements taught separately from form and practiced individually (not connected)
   b. All nine movements connected with transitions

As you can see, this is just a simple outline of the main content to be included in the course. At this stage, we aren't worried about being too detailed. We just want the highlights of what we'll cover in the course.

Course Description

Finally, as a last step in your blueprint, you'll want to put together a simple course description.

Your course description will include your ULP, plus some action-oriented bullet points that speak <u>directly</u> to your ideal student.

In other words, this description is <u>not</u> about the course content or the outline you just created. Instead, it's a statement about the major benefits the ideal student will get from this course.

Let me give you a real-life example of this type of course description from my own programs. As I've mentioned before, I teach a *Qi Masters* group of students, instructors, and masters. Our members are interested in more in-depth exploration of what it takes to be a master.

When I started this group, here were the ULP and the course description I wrote for my blueprint:

ULP:

Discover the Secrets to Becoming a "Qi Master" ...

How to Break Through to Higher Levels of Health, Stress Relief, Vitality, Energy, and Power in your Tai Chi and Qigong Practice

Course Description:

Discover our most effective secrets to...

- **Break through when you've "plateaued" and are stuck at your current level of Qi Development...**

- **Motivate yourself for "deeper" practice and obtain consistent "master level" results in your practice and teaching of Tai Chi and Qigong...**

- **Leap up several levels in your understanding and ability of both theory and application of advanced Qi skills...**

- **Explore the psychological, emotional, and spiritual aspects of becoming a master ... not sometime in the future, but RIGHT NOW...**

A three-time Hall of Fame Master is holding nothing back as he shows the secrets of Qi mastery to students and instructors who qualify for this training.

That is the ULP and course description that I wrote during my blueprinting stage. As you can see, this description is written directly to my ideal student avatar. It focuses on the benefits to the members of *Qi Masters*, not on the actual program's content.

Interestingly, when it came time to write a web page to promote the course, I simply used the ULP as the headline on the page. Then I put the course description as sub-headlines right below the headline. The rest of the page detailed the offer.

You can see that here:

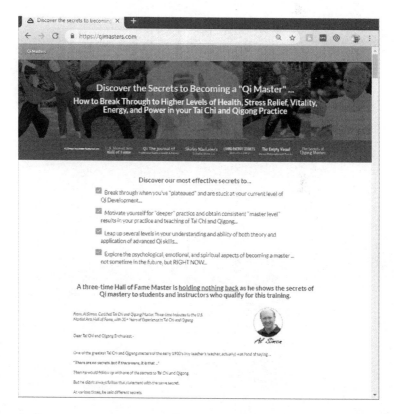

Once you have your basic blueprint, you can then move on to the third stage of the new course development process, the *pricing strategy* stage.

Develop Your Pricing Strategy

Pricing your course correctly involves a number of different factors. But for our purposes here in this book, let's focus on how pricing touches both student attraction and retention.

Pricing Works Like Your ULP

Pricing strategy is often neglected by Tai Chi and Qigong teachers, but it is an important part of attraction and retention.

Certainly, the Zero Drop Outs Strategy we learned in the first part of this book contains the most important steps.

But after *niche, avatar, location, offer,* **and ULP, the next most important factor in your success will be your** *pricing strategy.*

When it comes to pricing your classes, you'll find that a good pricing strategy works much like your ULP. It identifies students that are right for your class, but it also weeds out students who are wrong for your class.

You see, when you follow the Zero Drop Outs Strategy, you will be offering something special to your niche. If your niche has a difficult problem – one they are having trouble finding solutions for – they will pay you just about anything for your solution.

Well ... they'll pay <u>almost</u> anything. There are some limitations. But in general, if you are providing a strong offer and ULP to your niche, then serious students will understand the value of the solutions you offer. They'll also be willing to pay a fee that matches that value.

As a matter of fact, when you offer specialized solutions that match what your niche wants, the <u>wrong fee</u> will create attraction and retention problems. But the <u>correct fee</u> will actually <u>improve</u> both your attraction and retention.

Pricing Prevents Problems

Of course, it's obvious that you'll have <u>attraction</u> problems if your fee is <u>too high</u>. If you charge too much, your ideal students may not be able to afford it. But even if they could afford it, they may question its value if it's much higher than they expect. Either way, most won't sign up.

But let's say some do sign up, despite their uncertainty about the high price. They may then become <u>retention</u> problems. They may not stay around for follow-up classes if they feel like their first course with you didn't provide enough value to justify the high fee.

But in general, most teachers <u>don't</u> have attraction and retention problems from charging <u>too much</u>. They have problems from <u>charging too little</u>.

Remember our discussion of "the specialist vs. the generalist" when we talked about niching? We noted that people who specialize in more difficult problems generally have more authority and expert status than those who generalize. As part of that expert status, most people understand that high fees come with expertise and with high quality service.

Service providers who advertise cut-rate, bottom-dollar, low pricing are usually <u>not</u> thought of as providing high quality service.

Let's say you needed brain surgery, and you found a brain surgeon specializing in the particular problem you have. You then found out though that out of all the surgeons who operate on your particular problem, she had the cheapest fees of all brain surgeons. As a matter of fact, maybe she even promoted herself as the "low price" brain surgeon. Would you still use her as your surgeon?

There will always be penny pinchers in any niche that are looking for the best price. But when it comes to a health crisis such as brain surgery, most people don't want a low-cost surgeon. A low-cost surgeon might give them pause.

Pricing as an Indicator of Value

They might question the *lack of value* implied by the low fee. Generally, low fees imply low quality, so they may doubt that their "specialist" is actually all that "special." So instead, they'll want someone they are convinced will do the job right, and they'll be willing to pay more for the operation.

It's the same with just about every service field, including teaching Tai Chi and Qigong. There will be people for whom price is their number one concern. But for people who truly <u>want</u> and <u>need</u> a specialized service, a low fee will make them question the value, skills, and expertise of the so-called specialist.

Some people <u>say</u> they want the lowest price for everything the buy, but they don't actually mean it.

Very few people consistently wear the cheapest clothes, eat the cheapest food, drive the cheapest car, live in the cheapest house, use the cheapest cell phone (or no cell phone at all), or watch only free broadcast TV.

Instead, most people prioritize, saving money in certain areas, while spending more in other areas.

So if someone wants the cheapest Tai Chi or Qigong they can find, you've found someone that doesn't place a high value on learning Tai Chi or Qigong.

If you look at their lives, you'll often find they are prioritizing other wants and interests over tackling the problem they've come to you to solve.

They may be spending $1000 to have the latest smart phone, or $500 a year on streaming services to watch TV and movies, but they balk at the price you are asking for your Tai Chi and Qigong solution to their problem. In general, they want that phone or those streaming services more than they want their problem solved.

So if they balk at your fees, it shows their lack of commitment to solving the problems that you are offering to help them solve with Tai Chi or Qigong.

As professional instructors though, our fees reflect the specialized nature of what we teach.

One way to <u>undermine</u> your expert status is to charge <u>too little</u> for your courses, workshops, and programs.

Your fees should reflect the fact that you tackle tougher problems or harder-to-find curiosities than most instructors. If you are serious about providing your niche and ideal students with good quality instruction, offering them exactly what they want, your fees should reflect that.

What About Those Who Can't Afford It?

Of course, there will be people who just can't afford your course. They may want what you offer, but aren't in a good financial position. They aren't spending lavishly on non-essential items, but they still don't have the funds to pay for your course.

You will <u>always</u> find people who can't afford your course, no matter how low your price is.

I understand that some teachers feel uncomfortable when someone can't afford their courses. They may also feel reticent when asking for fees that reflect the actual value of the specialized nature of their teaching.

But you never have to feel badly when someone can't afford your teaching. Never. While your higher fees may stop prospective students from joining <u>your</u> class, they do <u>not</u> prevent them from learning Tai Chi or Qigong elsewhere.

Fortunately, these financially-strapped prospects have plenty of other opportunities for learning Qigong and Tai Chi besides your course.

As we've noted several times in this book, there are more teachers now than ever. Some of these teachers even provide low-cost or free options for price-conscious students. Students also have many video and online options, including many free ones. If they are truly interested in learning, they will find many ways that fit their budget.

Pricing Within Reason

Of course, there are times that you may want to teach low-cost or even free courses. There are right and wrong ways to go about that so that it doesn't undermine your expert authority. But as professional instructors, our fees for most of our teaching should reflect the specialized nature of what we teach. And most of your niche <u>will</u> be willing to pay ... *within reason.*

What do I mean by *within reason?*

For each niche, avatar, location, offer, and ULP, there is a target price range.

It's a range that realistically describes the lowest and highest possible prices that your ideal students will pay for your course, workshop, or program. If you price your course within this range, you will have <u>no problems</u> signing up your students in the niche, and keeping them motivated and coming back for more.

Attraction and retention problems will occur though if you price your course <u>outside</u> of this price range.

If you price your course <u>too high</u>, even your ideal students may not join. Pricing your course above this resistance price often creates *attraction* problems.

A <u>low</u> price, on the other hand, tends to create *retention* problems. With a low price, you'll often get less-than-ideal students registering, simply because the course is such a "great deal." But people who join your class simply because it's at a low price may not be fully committed to your niche, offer, and ULP. As a result, these less-than-fully-motivated students will easily drop out.

Determining the Correct Price Range

Most teachers go about pricing their courses by looking at what other teachers charge, or what similar courses cost, or even by looking at what they think other students want to pay or are willing to pay.

All of those are the <u>wrong</u> way to go about pricing your course. Using these incorrect pricing methods can undo all of the good "student attraction" work you've done in developing your niche, avatar, location, offer, and ULP.

I have a fool-proof method of pricing – one that supports your student attraction and retention goals. It's the method I use for pricing my courses, workshops, and programs. It's the method that has allowed me to sell over $1,000,000.00 (one million dollars) in Tai Chi and Qigong training.

This pricing strategy isn't difficult, but the details of how to go about it need some explaining. So to help you with pricing your course, I've created an online course on how to price your Tai Chi and Qigong programs.

The title of this online course is *"Attractive" Pricing for Tai Chi and Qigong: How to Get Students to Value Your Next Class or Workshop.*

In this course, we touch upon the strategic, practical, and psychological aspects of correct pricing for Tai Chi and Qigong.

We also discuss topics like pricing tiers for different types of students, plus the value of having guarantees for different types of programs.

We also cover the right and wrong ways to teach low-cost or free classes without creating attraction and retention problems.

But the bulk of the course is given over to showing you the exact method I use to determine the price for my courses, workshops, and programs. Over the course of five sessions, we cover in detail everything you need to help you determine the correct "student attraction and retention" price range for any program you teach.

The value of these five sessions to your success as Tai Chi and Qigong instructor is priceless.

To get access to this video series, just visit:

www.QiTeacher.com/price

Promoting Your Course

After you have your blueprint completed and your pricing strategy set, then it's time to start *promoting your course.*

Promoting your course is a huge topic, deserving of a book all to itself. But for the purposes of this book, let's look at how promotion affects both student attraction and retention.

When it comes to promoting your course, you'll need to:

- Develop your promotional strategy

- Develop your promotional communications

- Launch promotions and monitor for results

Strategy vs. Communications

When it comes to promotion and advertising, most teachers first think of the communications aspect of promotion.

In other words, they often look first to their *media* and their *message*.

By *media,* I mean the promotional channels they'll use. They'll look at options such as flyers, brochures, press releases, placements in publications like course catalogs, websites, social media posts, online text ads, etc.

By *message,* I mean the design and the contents of the promotion. The design is the way the promotion will look (the layout of the ad, flyer, brochure, website, post, etc.), and the contents are what the promotion actually says (the words and visuals used in the ad).

Of course, if you want a successful promotion, it's natural to want to spend time on what *media* you should use, the design of your *message,* and the contents of your *message.*

But when it comes to successful promotions, your *promotional strategy* is much more important than your *communications.*

Importance of List and Offer

By "promotional strategy," I'm referring to *who* you'll be targeting in your promotions, and *what* you'll be offering these people.

We call the *who* in this strategy your *list.* The *what* in this strategy is *your offer.*

Your *list* refers to the people you'll actually be putting your promotion in front of. This is the pool of prospective students that may be interested in joining your course, workshop, or program.

By *offer,* I'm referring to your course, workshop, and program.

Earlier in this book, we used the word *offer* to mainly refer to the title of your course, workshop, or program. We mean that here as well. But we are also including the benefits you'll be offering through your program, your *unique learning proposition* (ULP), and your pricing for the program.

All of that taken together is your promotional offer.

I know that a lot of people focus on *media* and *message* first when it comes to promoting their programs. The assumption is that if they have a well-designed flyer, brochure, website, social media page, etc., and if it says just the right things, students will register and sign up.

But it's usually not that simple. While *media* and *message* are important, *list* and *offer* are by far the more important factors.

List is actually the most important factor of them all. No matter how good your media and messages are, you have to put them in front of the right people. If you put it in front of people who aren't interested in what you offer, or who are interested but aren't in a position to take advantage of it, you'll have a hard time attracting students.

For example, if you are promoting a Qigong course geared towards seniors, it makes no sense to put your promotion in front of young martial artists. It doesn't matter how well-designed your promotional message is in that case. You are talking to the wrong group.

Offer is the second most important factor. Let's say you get in front of the right group, but you offer them a program that doesn't have clear benefits for them.

For example, let's say you want to reach seniors with your Qigong course, but you are offering them benefits like stress management, better creativity, improved learning, and increased productivity. Your offer of these "working person" benefits won't be of interest to a retired person.

List (the right people) and *offer* (the right course, benefits, and price) are clearly more important than having well-designed, well-written ads and promotions.

The Ground Work is Done

I would say that this should be your promotional priority: *list* first, then *offer,* then *media,* and lastly *message.* So you should focus on *list* and *offer* <u>first</u> when planning your promotions.

At this point though, when you are ready to plan your promotions, you've <u>already</u> laid some of the groundwork for *list* and *offer.*

If you've gone through the Zero Drop Outs Strategy in the first part of this book, you already have an idea of who should be on your list and what you should offer them.

The first three steps of the strategy - *niche, avatar,* and *location* - tell you <u>who</u> to put your offer in front of. The last two steps - your *offer/course title* and *ULP* – tell you <u>what</u> to put in front of them.

But let's go a little deeper into this concept of *list* for your promotions.

The Value of RWAs

For a successful promotion, you want to put your offer in front of <u>only</u> those prospective students that are "RWA."

"RWA" stands for "ready, willing, and able."

"Ready" means that the prospective student has the problem that your program solves, the need that it fulfills, or the curiosity that it satisfies. "Ready" also means that she is at that point in her life where your program makes sense to her. She's ready for it.

"Willing" means your prospective student is actively looking for a solution to his problem, or for something to fulfill his need or interest. And he will do just about anything to make that happen. He's not just "curious" or "interested." He's passionate about having his needs fulfilled in this area.

Now, he may not be fully aware that he's been doing it, but he has been actively looking for a course like yours or something just like it.

"Able" of course means that the prospective student is able to sign up for your program.

Obviously, she has to be able to afford it, but she also has to be at the point in her life where it makes sense to spend the money to get your solution. In addition, she has to be "able" in the sense that she has room in her schedule for your program, as well as a way to get to your program.

We call these people "RWA's" - the ready, willing, and able's. They are ready, willing, and able to take advantage of the solution and benefits provided by your offer.

The Power of the RWA List

Imagine you've created a new course, completed your blueprint, and set your pricing strategy. At this point, you are ready to promote the course.

But also imagine you don't have to worry about designing or posting flyers, or placing text ads online, or setting up social media pages to registrations.

Instead, you can fill your class just by sending out a few emails. Or maybe you can drop a few letters or postcards in the postal mail, and you start seeing sign-ups. Or maybe you can just make a few phone calls, or send a few text messages, and the registrations start pouring in.

That's the power of having your own RWA list.

If you have a list of RWAs, you don't have to struggle with distributing your message widely via flyers, ads, websites, or social media. You don't have to hope and pray that RWAs stumble upon your message somewhere and decide to register from it.

Instead, with your own list of RWAs, you can contact the ideal prospects for your new course directly.

Imagine how much time, energy, and money you'll save if you put your message in front of people you know are already right for it.

Building Your In-House RWA List

One of your main promotional tasks, as a Tai Chi or Qigong instructor, is to develop your own "in house" RWA list. This is a list of people who've expressed interest in the "niche solutions" you're providing now or that you've provided in the past.

You should have an in-house RWA list for each niche you teach in.

This list should include their name, of course, plus some method of contacting them – email address, physical address, phone number, text message number, etc.

How do you build this list?

First of all, your list should include all of the past students who've taken any niche-related courses, programs, or workshops you've already held.

Since these people have already shown they are RWA with their past registrations, they will often be enthusiastic for new programs you create.

You could also include on this list people who've inquired about your niche programs, but haven't been students yet.

If they've called, emailed, or messaged you to ask about your courses, they could be added to the list even if they didn't register. But you shouldn't just automatically add inquirers like this to the list. You should add them only if you believe they would be good prospective students.

Also, for these inquirers, you should ask them if they'd like to be added to your list.

When they email or call, just ask, "Can I add you to my list of interested students? That way, I can let you know whenever I have new programs for *[seniors, martial artists, cancer patients, stress management, or whatever their niche interest is]."*

By the way, you should also remove people from the list whenever they ask you to, or whenever you think they are no longer good prospective students. If it looks like their interest in the niche or in your offerings has dropped, you can remove them from the list.

Size Doesn't Matter

You'll soon learn that size of your RWA list doesn't matter. You don't need a large list for your promotions if everyone on your list is ready, willing, and able.

At one time, I had large prospect lists, especially for my online programs. I would send out regular promotions to lists of 30,000 to 50,000 people.

These days though, all of my RWA lists in all of my niches have less than 2,000 people. In some niches, the list is under 100 people. Yet, I still regularly hit the minimum numbers in my promotions, and I often hit the maximum.

Building smaller, more selective lists always results in better promotions. That's because you are focusing on

the real potential students. **You aren't wasting time and money on people who can't, won't, or don't register.**

Having a small list of just RWA's means you can focus on giving the best quality Tai Chi and Qigong programs you can to those who can, will, and do register.

Especially in a large niche, if you focus on trying to promote to *anyone* you can in the niche, you can lose time, money and energy before your course gets off the ground.

But if you focus on the RWA's, you can find new students even in the smallest niches.

But What If I'm Just Starting?

Obviously, if you are just starting as a teacher, you won't have a list of past students to start with. You also may not have had any inquiries yet, if this is the first course you've offered to your niche.

So you'll have to start from scratch building your list.

In that case, you may have to go the "broadcast" route to get your new students. By "broadcasting your message," I'm referring to getting your promotion widely distributed to a bunch of people. Of course, if your message gets in front of a lot of people, most of them won't be interested in it. But you're hoping that your ideal students are among this group and will stumble upon your message.

If you have to broadcast your message, you'll have to use more standard methods of promotions, such as flyers, brochures, listings in course catalogs, online ad sites (free and paid), social media advertising, press releases, etc.

While you often can't control who sees your broadcast message, some broadcast methods do give you the option of "targeting" your promotion to certain groups of people.

For example, most online ad services allow you to target your ads to specific physical locations. If you are an in-person teacher or coach, you can make sure your promotional ads are only shown to those who live in the area you defined in your location research. Again, many of these people won't be interested in your classes, but at least you won't be wasting money on advertising to those outside of your area.

Or if you are using offline advertising, you can make sure your flyers and brochures are located in places where your target prospects are likely to be.

It's also possible, at least in some online ads, to target people who have an interest in your niche. You can sometimes get really specific with this targeting.

For example, if you teach Tai Chi for cancer recovery in Portland, Oregon, you can sometimes set your ad to display only to *people in Portland, Oregon who have liked social media posts about Tai Chi and have visited websites on surviving cancer.*

That kind of targeting improves the odds of your broadcast message hitting your ideal prospects. Of course, a lot of non-RWA's will still see the message, but at least it improves the odds a bit.

While your ultimate goal for these ads is to get people to register for your course or program, keep in mind your first task should be to capture their contact information.

When you first talk, email, or message them, and they seem interested, get their contact information, and ask them if you can add them to your list of interested students. That way, even if they don't register, you've started building your list.

Broadcast Promotions at the Facility

If you are starting from scratch, here are some ideas for "broadcast" methods to build your list.

First of all, if you are teaching at a facility, see if the facility will aid you in your promotions.

If they produce a brochure or catalog, ask if your course could be listed there. If they have bulletin boards, ask if you can post a flyer or brochures. Also try to post flyers or brochures around the registration desk.

If they send regular email to their members (e.g., newsletters), ask if you can write a short blurb for it. Or ask if they'll send a solo email about your program to their members. If they have a postal list of their members, ask if you can pay to do a postal mailing to that list. Or if they will do a postal mailing on your behalf, announcing your program as their newest offering.

By the way, always offer to ghost-write these emails or postal mail pieces for them. Also offer to pay for the cost of the mailings. Most facilities will be more amenable to doing that if you are picking up the tab for printing and postage.

One word of warning, though. While these facilities have in-house lists of their members, don't just automatically use their list as your in-house RWA list. In other words, just because someone is on a list at the facility, that doesn't mean they are automatically a good prospect for your program. So always email or mail to that list first, and then add those who respond or register to your own RWA list.

Ask if you can talk to the staff at the facility, or even do a single free session or demo for the staff. In that way, the staff will know about your program and do a better job of promoting it to their members.

Other Ideas for Broadcast Promotions

Beyond broadcasting at the facility, you can also send your offer using more traditional broadcast channels.

You might use online text ads, online videos, social media posts, blog posts, flyers, press releases, newspaper ads, or ads in relevant magazines and local publications.

Keep in mind, when you are broadcasting a promotional message like this, you'll be back a bit into the mode of kissing a lot of frogs to find your Tai Chi princes and princesses.

But it will help if you've done a good job defining your niche, ideal students, and location, and then making sure your ads convey that information. In that way, you'll cut down on responses from those who are only mildly curious. The responses you do get will be from those who are more serious.

Promotional Communications

It's a bit beyond our scope here to go into detail on how to create your media and message. There's an art to designing good ads and writing good promotional "copy" (that is, the text of your promotional messages).

As a result, many teachers find writing ads for their courses and workshops difficult. It can be intimidating having to sit down to a blank page and create a "student attraction" ad from scratch.

Or even worse, they wind up creating ineffective, "non-attracting" ads that look just like everyone else's:

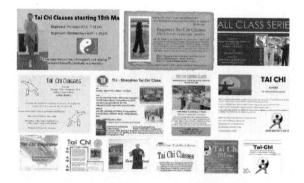

So to help you make sure **your ads** have "attractive" power, I have a resource for you. **I've created an online video presentation called** *Amazingly "Attractive" Ads for Tai Chi and Qigong: Five Ad Layouts to Fill Your Next Class or Workshop.*

In this video, I show how to use the full power of the *Zero Drop Outs* strategy in your ads to attract new students like a magnet.

This video shows you how to present your *offer* to your *list* in a way that serious students "get the message" about your teaching and respond to it.

I also show you <u>five easy layouts</u> to help you create these amazingly "attractive" ads.

The five layouts in this video make it easy to put together an amazing ad for your next class or workshop. You can use any one of these layouts as a printed flyer, brochure, or sales letter, or use it online on your website, in text ads, as a blog post, or as a social media post.

Every Tai Chi and Qigong instructor can use these ad layouts to get the most from their promotional efforts.

Since I want to see you succeed with your *Zero Drop Outs* strategy, I'm making this online presentation and these ad layouts <u>available for free</u> to anyone who has purchased this book.

You can download your copy of this video presentation plus the ad layout slides from this web page: <u>www.QiTeacher.com/bonuses</u>

Launching and Monitoring Results

Finally, once you have your promotional strategy and communications ready, then it's time to *launch your promotions*. This is where you get your ads and promotional material out in front of your prospective students.

Once your promotion is launched, you'll want to *monitor the results* to see how effective the promotion is at attracting prospects and converting them into students.

Based on what you see, you may need to adjust your strategy as you go along.

For example, while promoting a new course, I'll highlight different features or benefits at different times.

A certain ad, video, email, blog post, or flyer might highlight one specific benefit more than the others. I then might find that a lot of prospects register as a result of the promise of that particular benefit.

As a result, I may want to emphasize that benefit <u>more</u> during the rest of the promotional period.

Also, as new students register during the promotional period, I may ask them about what they are looking for from the course.

I'll then adjust my promotions if I find a number of students mentioning certain benefits they are looking for, especially if they are benefits that I hadn't included during my original research and planning.

For example, when I was first promoting my *Qi Masters* group, I created a "new members survey" that I sent to those who registered. In the survey, I asked them about the biggest challenges or roadblocks they faced to their progress in Tai Chi and Qigong. I also asked them what questions they had for me.

Some of the answers I received from these new members were on topics and benefits I hadn't originally included in my promotion. For example, motivation – both motivating themselves as well as motivating their students to practice – came up several times.

I hadn't previously thought about motivation as a major topic for the program. I had discussed motivation in other programs I'd taught in the past, but apparently my new members wanted to explore that topic even more.

So, since the topic fit in well with the *Qi Masters* group, I added it as a benefit to the promotional ads, emails, and videos I was using to attract members.

A number of prospective members subsequently registered when they found that this topic was to be part of the group's training material. That suggested that my niche and ideal students were still interested in the topic, even though we had covered them in a number of other programs.

You'll find that no matter how well you know a niche, there is still more to learn about its members.

The promotional period is a great time to learn about your own "blind spots" in the niche from your newly registered students.

When a Promotion Fails

Of course, <u>not</u> every promotion is successful. A certain number of your promotions will fail to reach the minimum number of registrations for your course.

These "failures" are important for two reasons.

First of all, you don't want to waste time teaching courses and programs that your ideal students *don't* want. In this way, a failed promotion allows you to let go of courses that your niche, location, and ideal students don't want.

But more importantly, these failures provide valuable information.

Failed promotions sometimes show you that you have misjudged the niche, the ideal student, or the location.

This is especially important when you are first entering a new niche. You may not actually have a good vision, a good idea, or a good feel for what the niche wants - even if you consider yourself part of the niche.

Our Zero Drop Outs Strategy is designed to help you with research and planning to reduce failed promotions, but each of us has our own blind spots in various niches.

However, as you continue to use these strategies, your knowledge of the niche will improve, and failed promotions are an important part of zeroing in on what a niche really wants.

Fortunately, the more you use the Zero Drop Outs Strategy, the better you become at knowing your niche and avatars, so your failures will become rarer.

When I first started out in my niches years ago, about seven out of every ten of my promotions did <u>not</u> attract the number of students I wanted.

But over time, as I became more skilled in the Zero Drop Outs Strategy, I got to know my niches better. I also became better skilled at creating student avatars and at doing location research.

These days, my promotional failures within a niche I know well are rare.

The Elusiveness of Timing

Here's one last bit of advice about failed promotions. Sometimes you can have the perfect niche, perfect avatar, perfect location, perfect offer, and perfect ULP – but the promotion still fails.

It fails not because your research was wrong, but because of *timing.*

Timing is one of those elusive factors that we don't always have control over, or even knowledge of.

You don't always know everything that is going on in your prospective students' lives. Work schedules, family situations, financial problems, and other outside factors might cause the ideal student to reject an offer this month that they might have been enthusiastic about last month or might immediately jump on next month.

I've often found that if I'm confident I have the right niche, avatar, location, offer, and ULP, but the promotion fails, I may try the promotion again at a future date. Often, the second time around, it will work.

I had one promotion I tried a few years back that received no registrations. Not a single one. So I cancelled the program and then forgot about it.

About two years afterwards, I stumbled across the files for the forgotten promotion on my computer when I was searching for something else. I decided to try the promotion again. I used the exact same niche, avatar, location, offer, ULP, blueprint, pricing, promotional strategy, and even the promotional communications. I used them just as they were, without any changes.

The promotion that had bombed two years earlier resulted in over one hundred registrations the second time around.

The whole point here is that monitoring the results of your promotions – positive or negative – can also provide you valuable feedback about your niche, ideal student, and location.

Once again we could do an entire book on promotion. But for right now, I want to make one last important point.

You should always do <u>your own</u> promotions for your courses, and not rely solely on others to promote them.

For example, I know some teachers hold classes at a martial arts school or at a health center, and they don't involve themselves in promotions. Instead, they rely exclusively on the school or center to find students for them.

That's a mistake.

You should do your own promotions, even if the school or center also promotes you. You will always be more motivated and dedicated to promoting yourself than anyone else will be.

Also, because you've done the research, you can better represent yourself and your courses, workshops, and programs. You will attract better students and be able to retain them better than if you rely on someone else's less-than-ideal promotion.

Creating Your Course

Once you have promoted your course, and you've met the minimum number of registrations needed to hold the course, it's time to *create the course.*

There's a lot that goes into creating your final course, especially if it's a book, video, or online program. Even if you teach in person, you still need to organize the material you'll be teaching into sessions.

But for the purposes of this book, let's just focus on a few aspects of course creation that touch upon student attraction and retention.

To create your course:

- Start with your blueprint and rough outline

- Adjust it based on results of your promotions

- Create a detailed session-by-session outline

- Create course material as needed.

You'll notice that we don't start creating the course until after we've completed our promotions and filled the class.

There are two important reasons for waiting to create the course until after the promotional step.

First of all, you don't want to do the work to create the course if you do not get the minimum number of students.

As we mentioned above in the promotional phase, you may find your promotion fails. That may indicate this course isn't right for this niche. So there's no point wasting time creating a course no one wants.

The second reason to wait to create your course is that you might want to make adjustments to the content based on what you learn during the promotion and registration period.

In the example I gave a few pages ago, I found out during one of my promotions for my *Qi Masters* group that my members wanted more on the topic of *motivation.* That topic wasn't in my original blueprint for the group.

By waiting until after the promotional period to create the training material, I was able to add that topic into the program, increasing its value to the group members.

So at this point in the course development process, you take the blueprint and rough outline you created earlier, and adjust it based on the results of your promotion. Then you would create a detailed session-by-session outline of the course.

After you have that outline, you would create any material you needed to deliver the course – teaching notes, student handouts, online videos and transcripts, a membership website, etc.

The end goal of this step is to get everything ready that you need to teach the course.

Just keep in mind – your final course <u>must</u> fulfill all the promises you made in your offer, your ULP, and your promotions.

It may seem obvious, but if you don't deliver what you've promised, you'll lose students rather quickly from the class.

More about that in our next step.

Delivering Your Course

The final step of the course creation process is to actually *deliver the course.*

This is where you start teaching if it's an in-person course, or you get the training materials into your students' hands if it's a remote learning course.

Course delivery is also a rather large topic. But let's focus on the aspects that touch upon our main themes in this book – student attraction and retention.

For the course delivery step you need to:

- Teach the course.

- Fulfill the promises of your offer, ULP, and promotions.

- Use a teaching model that supports these promises, especially the ULP.

- Use communication styles that reinforce the ULP.

- Make adjustments to course content based on working with students.

- Collect success stories and referrals.

What's absolutely the most important part of all of this is that you need to fulfill the promises made by your offer, your USP, and your promotions.

You should especially focus on the promises made in your ULP, because that's usually the primary benefits your students wanted when they signed up for the course.

In other words, you have to <u>deliver</u> at this point.

If you mentioned certain benefits or particular results that the students would get as part of your ULP, you <u>have to make sure</u> the course you teach provides those benefits and results.

I've often found that some of the benefits come easily from the course *contents* – that is what you are teaching. But more often than not, what really makes the difference here is the *teaching model* you use. In other words, the benefits come more from *how* you are teaching rather than *what* you are teaching.

The teaching model you use has to support the promises you've made in your offer, ULP, and promotions.

As part of the teaching model, this is also where tools like *communication styles* come in handy. You want to use styles that further reinforce the ULP in the minds of your students.

While you are teaching, you will also probably make adjustments to the course content. So even though you've blueprinted the course in an early phase and you created the session-by-session outlin in the previous phase, you still might change the course during the delivery phase.

Especially for in-person courses, as you are working with your students, you'll find out more about what they're interested in. You may even wind up going in unexpected directions at times, based on their interests. So you may want to adjust the course content as you go along, to satisfy those interests. (It's important that these unexpected directions are based on their interest, not your own self-indulgence.)

Finally, as part of the delivery process, you should also be collecting *success stories and referrals* from your students.

By *success stories,* I'm referring to testimonials anytime a student sees some results from your program. You need to collect that testimonial while you're delivering the course.

Also this is a great time to ask your students for referrals – that is, if they know of people who might also be interested in your course.

Asking your students to refer those people to you is a great way to get access to more potentially ideal students.

Think of it this way.

You already have a class that has a lot of your ideal students in it - or at least students that responded well to your ideal student avatar.

These students are probably friends with people that are *like them.*

In other words, their friends might also be close to your ideal student avatar.

So referrals are an important part of continuing to promote your course or program, especially if you'll be offering it more than once.

Congratulations

Congratulations on completing this book on *Zero Drop Outs: The Qi Masters Guide to Finding and Keeping Students in Tai Chi and Qigong.*

I hope that you now have a better understanding of the Zero Drop Outs Strategy you can use to fill your classes, workshops, and programs with dedicated, enthusiastic students, cut your drop-out rate to zero, and attract new students like a magnet.

We've covered a lot in this short book about what it takes to be a successful instructor. But if you would like to really boost your success both as a teacher and as a practitioner, you would benefit greatly from our *Qi Masters* program.

To help you explore more deeply into the physical, mental, emotional, and energetic aspects of becoming a master of Tai Chi and Qigong, please visit us online at **www.QiMasters.com.**

And thank you again for purchasing this book and supporting our work. We appreciate having dedicated instructors like you who show their support.

As always, you have my best wishes for success in Tai Chi, Qigong, and Chi Development.

Complimentary Bonuses Just For You (a $97 Value)

I have some special bonuses exclusively for you as a reader of *Zero Drop Outs: The Qi Masters Guide to Finding and Keeping Students in Tai Chi and Qigong.*

Just go online to www.QiTeacher.com/bonuses and you can download the following:

✓ **Step-by-Step *Zero Drop Outs* Planning Guide**

This downloadable, printable guide walks you through the Zero Drop Outs Strategy covered in this book.

Give yourself the power to attract, motivate, and keep new students with this short, handy Zero Drop Outs Strategy Planning Guide.

This guide will make sure you cover all five steps of the strategy to give you the maximum "student attraction" power. Use this guide to plan out your own classes, workshops, or programs.

✓ *Zero Drop Outs* **Planning Video**

Let me take you by the hand and walk you through your new Zero Drop Outs Planning Guide.

In this short online video, I'll take you step-by-step through the Planning Guide.

This video will show you exactly what you need to do to put the power of student attraction to work for you in your next class, workshop, or program.

It will help you make sure you are doing each student attraction step the right way.

As we go through them in this video, you'll make sure each step is in place and ready to go to make your next class a "student attraction success."

✓ **Amazingly "Attractive" Ads for Tai Chi and Qigong: Five Ad Layouts to Fill Your Next Class or Workshop (video)**

Many teachers find writing ads for their courses and workshops difficult. It can be intimidating having to sit down to a blank page and create a "student attraction" ad from scratch.

Or even worse, they wind up creating ineffective, "non-attracting" ads that look just like every other teacher's ads.

So to help you make sure the ads you create have "attractive" power, I have a resource for you.

I've created an online video presentation called *Amazingly "Attractive" Ads for Tai Chi and Qigong: Five Ad Layouts to Fill Your Next Class or Workshop.*

In this video, I show how to use the full power of the *Zero Drop Outs* strategy in your ads to attract new students like a magnet.

This video shows you how to present your *offer* to your *list* in a way that serious students "get the message" about your teaching and respond to it.

I also show you <u>five easy layouts</u> to help you create these amazingly "attractive" ads.

The five layouts in this video make it easy to put together an amazing ad for your next class or workshop. You can use any one of these layouts as a printed flyer, brochure, or sales letter, or use it online on your website, in text ads, as a blog post, or as a social media post.

Every Tai Chi and Qigong instructor can use these ad layouts to get the most from their promotional efforts.

Since I want to see you succeed with your *Zero Drop Outs* strategy, I'm making this online presentation and these ad layouts <u>available for free</u> to anyone who has purchased this book.

You can download all of these special bonuses online from this web page: <u>www.QiTeacher.com/bonuses</u>

I hope you'll accept these bonuses as my thank you for reading this book. It's one of the ways I go the extra mile to show my appreciation for your support.

As always, I wish you the best for your qi practice and teaching.

Al J. Simon

Special Resource: *"Attractive"* Pricing for Tai Chi and Qigong

Here's another special resource for readers of *Zero Drop Outs.*

Pricing strategy is often neglected by Tai Chi and Qigong teachers, but it is an important part of attraction and retention.

Most teachers go about pricing their courses by looking at what other teachers charge, or what similar courses cost, or even by looking at what they think other students want to pay or are willing to pay.

All of those are the wrong way to go about pricing your course. Using these incorrect pricing methods can undo all of the good "student attraction" work you've done in developing your *Zero Drop Outs* strategy.

You see, for each niche, avatar, location, offer, and ULP, there is a *target price range*.

It's a range that realistically describes the lowest and highest possible prices that your ideal students will pay for your course, workshop, or program. If you price your course within this range, you will have <u>no problems</u> signing up your students in the niche, and keeping them motivated and coming back for more.

Attraction and retention problems will occur though if you price your course <u>outside</u> of this price range.

So how do you determine that price range for any class, workshop, or program you might offer?

I have a fool-proof method of pricing. It's the method I use for pricing my courses, workshops, and programs. It's the method that has allowed me to sell over $1,000,000.00 (one million dollars) in Tai Chi and Qigong training.

This pricing strategy isn't difficult, but the details of how to go about it need some explaining. So to help you with pricing your course, I've created an online course on how to price your Tai Chi and Qigong programs.

The title of this course is *"Attractive" Pricing for Tai Chi and Qigong: How to Get Students to Value Your Next Class or Workshop.*

In this course, we touch upon the strategic, practical, and psychological aspects of correct pricing for Tai Chi and Qigong.

We also discuss topics like pricing tiers for different types of students, plus the value of having guarantees for different types of programs.

We also cover the right and wrong ways to teach low-cost or free classes without creating attraction and retention problems.

But the bulk of the course is given over to showing you the <u>exact method</u> I use to determine the price for my courses, workshops, and programs.

Over the course of five short sessions, we cover in detail everything you need to help you determine the correct "student attraction and retention" price range for any program you teach.

Each online session is available as a video presentation, an audio presentation, and a written transcript. You get all three versions with your course. So you can watch, listen, or read – whichever way you learn best – or do all three.

The value of these five sessions to your success as a Tai Chi and Qigong instructor is priceless.

To get access to this video series, just go online and visit:

www.QiTeacher.com/price

Al J. Simon

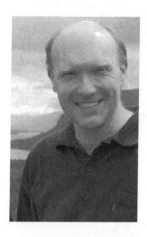

About the Author

Al Simon is a certified Tai Chi and Qigong master. He is the "founding father" of online Tai Chi and Qigong instruction. He was the first master to teach online in 2003, and he now has 4,500 online students all over the world. Online sales of his Tai Chi and Qigong programs have topped over $1,000,000.00 (one million dollars).

Al Simon learned his first Qigong exercises in 1975. He studied Zen meditation in 1982 and began Tai Chi in 1984. He received certification from Master Lawrence Galante, author of the book *Tai Chi - The Supreme Ultimate*. Al is also mentioned in the book *Mastering Yang Style Tai Chi.*

Al has been inducted into the United States Martial Arts Hall of Fame three times. Al was inducted with the **rank of "Master"** by the International Martial Arts Headfounders Grandmasters Council. He was also inducted with the **rank of "Founder"** for the development of the ChiFusion™ Tai Chi and Qigong program.

Al is also the author of the eleven books, including *50 True Chi Stories; To Float Like Clouds, To Flow Like Water; Three Monk Mindfulness; Qigong Self-Massage and Chi Washing;* and *The Four Treasures of Tai Chi and Qigong.*

Al appeared as a guest on both season one and season two of the *Living Energy Secrets* series, as well as BlogTalk Radio's *Secrets of Qigong Masters.* In addition, Al's articles on Tai Chi, Qigong, and Chi Development have appeared in publications such as *Wholistic Alternatives, Natural Health Newsletter, The Empty Vessel,* and *Chi Journal.* His Chi Development program was also spotlighted on Shirley MacLaine's *Independent Expression Radio* show.

Al is also a member of Mensa, the high I.Q. society.

Your Invitation

Want to become a more successful Tai Chi or Qigong instructor, while at the same time learning more advanced material you can teach your students?

We invite you to join us as we explore how to break through to higher levels of health, stress relief, vitality, energy, and power in your Qi teaching and practice.

For support in taking the next steps towards higher levels in your teaching and practice, please visit us online at:

www.QiMasters.com

Made in the USA
Lexington, KY
29 October 2019